AF446442

The Superfood Prescription: Refuel Your Mind & Body

100 Supercharged Foods to Revitalize & Transform Your Health

Chrío Zoë

First published by Zoë Publishing 2023

Copyright © 2023 by Chrío Zoë

All rights reserved. No part of this publication may be reproduced, stored or transmitted in any form or by any means, electronic, mechanical, photocopying, recording, scanning, or otherwise without written permission from the publisher. It is illegal to copy this book, post it to a website, or distribute it by any other means without permission.

Chrío Zoë asserts the moral right to be identified as the author of this work.

Chrío Zoë has no responsibility for the persistence or accuracy of URLs for external or third-party Internet Websites referred to in this publication and does not guarantee that any content on such Websites is, or will remain, accurate or appropriate.

Designations used by companies to distinguish their products are often claimed as trademarks. All brand names and product names used in this book and on its cover are trade names, service marks, trademarks and registered trademarks of their respective owners. The publishers and the book are not associated with any product or vendor mentioned in this book. None of the companies referenced within the book have endorsed the book.

Legal Notice:

Under no circumstances will any blame or legal responsibility be held against the publisher, or author, for any damages, reparation, or monetary loss due to the information contained within this book, including, but not limited to, errors, omissions, or inaccuracies. either directly or indirectly.

This book is copyright protected. It is only for personal use. You cannot amend, distribute, sell, use, quote or paraphrase any part, or the content within this book, without the consent of the author or publisher.

Disclaimer Notice:

Please note the information contained within this document is for educational and entertainment purposes only. All effort has been executed to present accurate, up to date, reliable, complete information. No warranties of any kind are declared or implied. Readers acknowledge that the author is not engaged in the rendering of legal, financial, medical or professional advice. The content within this book has been derived from various sources. Please consult a licensed professional before attempting any techniques outlined in this book. Book

First edition

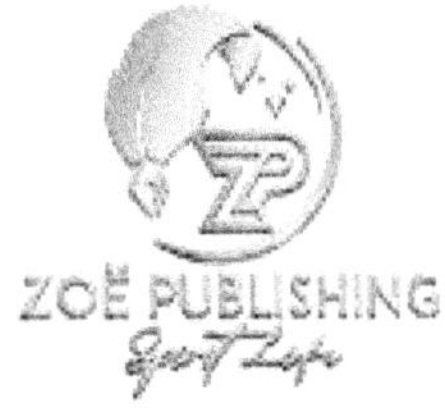

Medical Disclaimer

For those of you who are seeking personal medical advice, please ensure that you consult with a certified medical professional. The information that I am providing should not be used for any form of diagnosis or treatment of any illness, health complications, or underlying medical issues. If you are under the impression that you are dealing with a medical affliction, you should never self-diagnose. When dealing with a medical issue, I advise all of you that you should always consult with your physician or any other licensed healthcare professional.

Acknowledgement

Writing this book has been a labor and a journey that I couldn't have undertaken without the incredible support and encouragement of many individuals. I am profoundly grateful to all those who have played a part in bringing this project to fruition.

I would like to thank each person who was instrumental in shaping my path to writing this manuscript. My sincerest appreciation goes to the countless friends and family who graciously gave me space and time to make this book become a reality.

First and foremost, I want to express my deepest gratitude to my family whose unwavering belief in me and constant encouragement have been my driving force. Your love and support have sustained me through the challenges of this creative process. I give honor to my late parents, Stephen and Pearl, whose unwavering belief has been the catalyst to propel me in this journey. Their constant encouragement and unconditional love have been my strength to pursue this endeavor. I say thank you to my siblings Michael, Anthony, Pauline and Sharon who have now passed on but are the silent voices that ignited me to write this book. Through their life, in their own small contributing way, I have come to realize that this journey we call life is valuable and how we start the journey does not dictate how we finish it.

I would like to thank all of my mentors and teachers who helped me by sharing their invaluable knowledge base with me, as they guided me from a place of knowing in shaping my ideas and refining my writing. I cherish your warm guidance, encouragement, and belief in me, and my potential and I can attest to the fact that it has been transformative. I am sincerely hoping that this book will serve as a helpful resource and companion guide on my readers' journey toward self-improvement, empowerment, and fulfillment.

I'd also like to thank the team at AIA and Publishing Services for their dedication and hard work in bringing this book to life. Your expertise coaching and guidance in outlining, design, formatting, and marketing have been pivotal in turning my manuscript into a polished publication.

Additionally, I am grateful to my dear friends, who provided much-needed moral support and encouragement during the writing process. I am forever grateful for your influence and for your push to encourage me into what you believe I could be. Thank you all for the guidance and the wisdom you shared with me as I stumbled along my sometimes-rocky road of personal growth and self-discovery. I extend my heartfelt appreciation to my friends and colleagues who provided valuable feedback, engaged in insightful discussions, and cheered me on during moments of doubt. Your enthusiasm has been contagious and uplifting.

Finally, I want to acknowledge my readers—those who will engage with this book. Your curiosity and interest in my ideas fuel my passion for writing, and I hope this book resonates with you in meaningful ways. In writing this book, I've come to realize that the journey is made sweeter by the presence of supportive souls. To all those I've mentioned and to anyone whose name might have been inadvertently omitted, please know that your impact has been immeasurable.

To all of you, your enthusiasm, engagement, and support to me have been more than appreciated. Let me end by saying once again to my readers that I applaud you for buying this book to enhance and empower your personal development. I trust that this book will meet your desire.

With heartfelt thanks,

Chrío Zoë

Contents

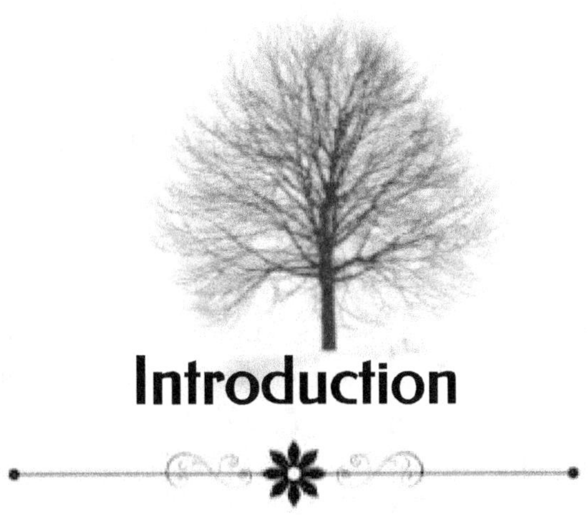

Introduction

You don't have to eat less, you just have to eat right.

–Unknown

When a person sees the word super, it gives them a great feeling or sparks their interest in finding out what it is about an item or product that makes it super. When you were younger, your teacher and/ or parents told you that you did a "superb job!" You felt amazing, and it boosted your confidence level and drive. Most of us have a love for superheroes and wish that we had their super abilities. Think about it for a second: The word super is tied to greatness. Human beings will naturally gravitate towards things that are super and anything that can increase their longevity and improve their health. However, despite how many people love the idea of living longer and improving their health and are intrigued by anything with super in front of it.

The truth is, if some of you were Superman or Superwoman, healthy foods would be your kryptonite. There are many of you who struggle with being consistent with making healthy choices when it comes to food and exercise. It is not that you do not want to; it is remaining consistent that is the issue, and for some of you, you are not patient with yourselves and want a quick fix and immediate results. In some cases, you set unrealistic goals for yourself, and when they do not happen, you feel as if you have failed or are not good enough. However, the reality is that what you set out for yourself was not achievable in the time frame that you set. What I want those of you who are reading this to know is that struggling with maintaining a healthy lifestyle does not make you a bad person and that you are not alone. Also, there are some of you who have received misinformation as it pertains to certain foods and health, and there are some of you who may not have received that much information at all. This is why I felt the need to shed some light on superfoods and what you can do to recharge your body and mind. Along with providing tips on being consistent, if you stumble during this new change in your life, all that matters is that you get up and go at it again.

When it comes to food, there are no strict requirements that a food must fulfill in order to be classified as a superfood; these foods are not going to a job interview. Nevertheless, they are not a nutritionally established group of foods. However, the term is usually reserved for whole meals that are particularly high in nutrients and often low in calories. Superfoods improve your immunity and lower the risk of illness development or progression, which contributes to your overall health promotion.

Although the nutritional qualities of each superfood differ, they are often connected to:

- Increase in heart wellness

- A robust immune system

- Prevention of cancer

- Lowering your level of inflammation

- Reduction in cholesterol levels

Superfoods deserve to have the word super placed before them, as they are a set of foods that are super-healthy. But it should be highlighted that not every healthy food that you may be consuming falls in the superfood slot. Superfoods are the ones that offer exceptional health benefits beyond what their nutritional composition may suggest.

Reading that line alone should pique your interest even more. Superfoods are typically abundant in:

- **Antioxidants**: They are shields, as they are excellent for your body to have because they protect your cells from damage and reduce your risk of heart disease, cancer, and other illnesses, diseases, and disorders.

- **Minerals**: Your body flourishes when necessary nutrients—like calcium, potassium, iron, and the like—are present.

- **Vitamins**: Rather than having to set your phone's reminder to take supplements, wouldn't it be better to obtain these organic substances from nutritious foods like superfoods? Because, let's be honest, there are times that you forget to check your reminders.

It should be noted that superfoods tend to have a higher level of:

- **Fiber**: Fiber aids in the control of blood sugar in Type 2 diabetes; it also plays a huge part in the prevention of heart disease and cholesterol reduction.

- **Flavonoids**: Plant-based flavonoids, which were once called vitamin P, have anti-inflammatory and anti-carcinogenic qualities.

- **Healthy fats**: No one is a fan of the word fat; however, there are healthy fats, also referred to as "good fats." Monounsaturated and polyunsaturated fats help decrease cholesterol and stave off heart disease and stroke.

Our bodies need fuel; when it is not being fueled properly, it does not function well, and that can be problematic. Having a healthy, nutrient-rich lifestyle does wonders for your body, as it gives your body the fuel it needs, helps your muscles, and does wonders for your mind. There are many people who are not getting enough nutrients; most of us are not consuming enough vitamins, minerals, and antioxidants, and having that shortage has us not performing and/or looking our best. So, how do you correct this?

I will delve into various nutrient-dense foods that you can make a part of your life that will improve your body, as I want you all to live your best life. Some nutrient-rich foods include:

- Vegetables

- Fruits

- Whole grains and whole-grain products

- Fat-free or low-fat dairy products

- Seafood

- Chicken and other lean meats

- Eggs

- Legumes, such as beans and peas

- Nuts and seeds

Keep in mind that the ingredients on this list are whole foods. Ideally, you should prioritize minimally processed foods while consuming nutrient-rich foods. These foods become less nutrient-rich and more calorie-dense after processing (for example, by adding fats, sugars, etc.), which will defeat the purpose. Increasing your consumption of the nutrient-rich foods listed above will have a positive impact on your health.

There are a number of foods that are nutrient-rich that are great for you to incorporate into your diet, and they are:

- **Whole grains**: Millet, sorghum, and quinoa

- **Vegetables**: Roots and tubers, such as sweet potatoes, which are great for you, and lovely dark green leafy vegetables like spinach or kale

- **Dairy**: Yogurt and cheese, in moderation.

- **Seafood**: This includes tasty salmon and other omega-3-rich fish, as well as shellfish like clams or mussels. If you are allergic to shellfish, this does not apply to you, but you can include fish if you are also free from this allergy.

- **Meats**: Chicken, pork, and organ meats (e.g., beef liver) are rich in iron and are great for people who suffer from iron deficiency and anemia.

- **Nutrient-rich**: Do not forget fruits! Mango, grapefruit, cantaloupe, and other vitamin A-rich fruits

What Are the Benefits of Consuming Superfoods?

I have to take this time to also include what the benefits of consuming superfoods are. Consuming these superfoods will do your entire body good.

1. **Consuming superfoods will do wonders for your heart**: In Chapter 2, I will go into details about what kinds of superfoods are linked to heart improvement. But for now, I will say that those superfoods will assist in maintaining healthy blood pressure, lowering cholesterol, and reducing inflammation, all of which will minimize the probability of cardiovascular diseases.

2. **Weight management**: Many of us are all about having that summer body. However, it is also important to manage and maintain a healthy weight. Superfoods can be very helpful to people who are simply trying to control their weight. In addition to being high in fiber and low in calories, it can help with weight loss or maintenance by promoting feelings of fullness, which will not leave room for overeating.

3. **Cognitive function**: Your brain is the most beautiful thing that you possess. It stores memories, helps with learning new skills, etc. It is top tier, and many of us are all about protecting it. Certain superfoods, like leafy greens and blueberries, contain components that can enhance cognitive function and fend off aging-related cognitive decline. These superfoods may enhance focus and memory while also promoting brain health.

4. **Digestive health**: There are certain superfoods, like chia seeds, that can support a healthy digestive tract microbiome. Immunity, emotional

modulation, and better digestion are all linked to a balanced intestinal ecosystem.

5. **Skin health**: Who doesn't love a great skin glow? Superfoods that are high in vitamins and good fats, like avocados, play a huge role in maintaining healthy, glowing skin. Superfoods can assist in enhancing skin texture and lessening the appearance of aging. Let us be honest, the idea of looking forever young is quite appealing.

6. **Disease prevention**: The main thing I want to stress is that your health is important, along with longevity. By consuming a range of superfoods, you can lower the chance of developing chronic illnesses such as diabetes, some types of cancer, and neurological disorders. These superfoods' dietary components can improve your general health and fortify your immune system.

7. **Energy boost**: Lacking energy lately? The truth is, not many people want to drink energy drinks all the time, and they are also packed with sugar! Superfoods provide an organic energy source without the energy crashes that are frequently associated with caffeine or other sugary snacks. Isn't it great to get an energy boost and be healthy? These superfoods give you a steady stream of energy that keeps you focused and engaged throughout the whole day.

8. **Detoxification**: There are certain superfoods, like cruciferous vegetables (broccoli, kale, etc.), that

possess ingredients that help the body's biological detoxification process by supporting the elimination of dangerous pollutants.

What Are the Benefits of Eating Nutrient-Rich Foods?

The goal that most of you should be aiming for is to eat clean. When you eat a clean, nutrient-rich diet, it will be beneficial for your overall health, especially as you get older. The risk of a nutritional deficiency is higher in seniors than in other age groups. Including more nutrient-rich foods in your day-to-day eating comes with great benefits, such as:

- Greater nutritional content per calorie. That will help you maintain a healthy weight. Always remember that balance is key.

- Lower your chances of major health issues associated with age and nutritional deficits, such as lowering your risk of osteoporosis, anemia, and cognitive decline.

- Better-quality sleep.

- A vast improvement in your overall mood and psychological well-being.

- Improved muscle strength comes with various advantages for seniors, such as lowering your chance of accidents and falls.

🌱 More mobility and flexibility, as well as better joint health.

Nutrition is an important aspect of your health and wellness, and many of you struggle with keeping healthy and giving your body what it needs. For some of you, it is easy to gravitate towards snacks (e.g., ice cream, potato chips, chocolate, nachos, fries, and variations of fries that are loaded with cheese and bacon, etc.) because they are tasty and give you a level of comfort; however, there is no balance. Those "tasty" high-calorie, salty snacks are getting more attention than fruits and vegetables, and that imbalance is not good for your body. This is your body, and you must take care of it. We cannot reboot and/or trade our bodies for new ones. The idea may seem appealing, but it just cannot happen. There are not many things in life we have control over, but our health and fitness are things that we are masters of.

You may be wondering why you should even take my research, advice, and knowledge into consideration. You may have watched a lot of medical shows; maybe even someone in your family told you that you are getting a bit "chubby" and need to shed a few pounds, and they are sharing information that has not been beneficial. So, what makes me any different? Well, I would like to take this time to introduce myself.

About the Author

Being over 60, I am very passionate about securing vitality through a healthy lifestyle. I am not just a proponent of a healthy lifestyle; I am a living testament to its transformative power. My journey is more than just a physical transformation; it's a holistic approach that encompasses mind, body, and spirit. With unwavering dedication, I have embraced a lifestyle that prioritizes self-care, mindful choices, and a commitment to nourishing my body from the inside out.

As I grew older over the years, my health became a major concern that I could no longer ignore. I suffered a massive stroke because of bad eating habits, which flooded my system with too many of the wrong foods that did not do my body or health any good. During that time, I was on medication, but I could not stand the fact that I'd be taking it for the rest of my life!

I had to make a decision: Either I continue living on various medications and junk food, or I teach myself that either I control food or food controls me. It was there and then that it became obvious that I invested in food that was not only "right" but had the potential to have a positive impact on my health and longevity.

Even though I live with the residuals of my stroke daily, I am not complaining because it's truly a miracle for me to still be alive and be able to intimately guide others so that they may avoid the setbacks I had to deal with.

I am dedicated to educating folks like you who are living the way I once lived. You have a desire to eat clean and have developed a deep dedication to what goes into your body; however, you just don't know where to start.

I don't just speak or read about what it means to use food as medication; I live that lifestyle and consume healthy food daily, and because of that, I am enjoying the results of my unwavering dedication and discipline. Once I started on my journey of incorporating superfoods into my diet and eating clean, I went from 200 pounds to 155 pounds and have maintained this for the last ten years.

I have written this book for you using extensive research, my experience, and my knowledge to ensure that you don't have to go a day further wondering what you can do to achieve your health goals and start feeling good about your body again. The information I have for you in this book has worked for me, and I am confident that with discipline and the same passion that drove you to read this far, it is seamlessly going to work for you too!

Are you ready to revitalize and transform your health? Then let's get started!

Chapter 1

Unlocking Your Body's True Potential by Understanding Superfoods

Your diet is a bank account. Good food choices are good investments.

–Bethenny Frankel

I wish I could give you a magical potion that will give you specific superhero features of your favorite Marvel or DC superhero. The idea sounds great, I know. However, this does not mean you cannot reach your full potential nutrition-wise, and that within itself is superhero energy. The aim is to understand what you need to consume and the benefits that will keep your body performing at its maximum capacity. Including these foods in your life will give your body a great chance at warding off illnesses and being able to function better if there is a mild illness that you are currently dealing with. Some of you may be reading this and wondering if there is any real truth behind it. I know it will take more than how I structure my words to convince you about this topic; you will want more information. Don't worry. I will be diving deep into the matter, so grab your scuba gear and take a dive with me.

The term superfoods have become popular in recent times, but I want to let you know that the term can be documented dating all the way back to the turn of the twentieth century. If any one of you were to take out your mobile device or laptop and google the word superfood, you would see close to ten million results. Yes, I said ten million results (*What are superfoods and are they really super?*, 2012). There are a variety of articles out there on this topic. There are people who have a deep-rooted passion for nutrition and have written blogs dedicated to this topic, along with corporations that supply nutritional supplements that share information online. Superfoods, overall, are defined as foods, particularly fruits and vegetables, whose nutritional value offers a health advantage over other types of food.

For the most part, human beings value information that can support these findings. There are many things that we have been told are great for us, but later, we found out they were not. Separating fact from fiction, or rather, hype, is important. Scientific evidence is a great place to start. Not only are blueberries tasty, but they have been tested to see what makes them a superfood. Not only is it more well-known and well-liked, but blueberries have been the subject of numerous studies by researchers interested in their potential health benefits. It has been observed that the high amounts of antioxidant plant components found in berries, particularly those referred to as anthocyanins, both stop the growth and eliminate malignant human colon cells. There are more antioxidants found in blueberries that have been demonstrated to stop and even reverse age-related memory loss in mice. Antioxidants are chemicals that stave off dangerous free radicals from entering the body's cells. Free radicals are substances that are not only produced naturally by the body during metabolism but also in things like alcohol and cigarette smoke. The body may experience oxidative stress due to an excess of free radicals, which can damage cells and result in chronic diseases like diabetes, heart disease, and cancer (*What are superfoods and are they really super?*, 2012).

Other fruits, such as pomegranates and acai berries, have also received the superfoods title, which, as you know, is a big deal. Strong antioxidant qualities have been demonstrated in acai berry fruit pulp. Pomegranate juice has been shown in studies to have the potential to lower blood pressure, and for people with hypertension, that is a huge benefit (the health benefits of superfoods will be discussed later on). However, another super quality of pomegranate juice is that, for healthy people, it can lessen oxidative stress in a short-term period. Both of them pose a serious risk for heart disease. Beetroot has also been touted as a heart-healthy superfood, much like pomegranate juice. The body is said to transform its high nitrate content into nitric oxide, which has been demonstrated to reduce blood pressure and the propensity for blood clotting in humans, among other things. Similar claims have been made about how cocoa reduces blood pressure and increases blood vessel flexibility to minimize the risk of heart disease. It is believed that the high concentration of flavonoid-containing chemicals in cocoa is to blame for this. Finally, there is a barrage of evidence that the omega-3 fatty acids in salmon and other oily fish may help prevent cardiac problems in high-risk people and reduce joint discomfort in rheumatoid arthritis sufferers. This has led to salmon being included on superfood lists on a regular basis.

Nutrient Density and Bioavailability Work Well Together

When you know what works for your body and what the best combination for you is, you will see improvements in your skin, health, and overall function of your body. Aging is inevitable; however, we all want to age well and gracefully and still maintain the capability to do certain things. Therefore, the change begins now. Consuming nutrient-dense food is a whole vibe. Not only does it prevent you from suffering from nutrient deficiencies, but it also helps prevent serious health issues later in life. While some of you may be aware of nutrient density, bioavailability gets lost in the group chat. Take for example, spinach. It is a great leafy food; it aids with weight loss, among other things, and it is packed with calcium. But here is the thing: calcium is not particularly bioavailable. What I plan to do for you is break down the two (nutrient density and bioavailability) and show you how they work well together. Let's get this show on the road!

Nutrient Density Does Your Body Good

The amount of healthy nutrients in a specific number of calories is how nutritional density is typically defined. Basically, what I am saying is that foods that are higher in beneficial nutrients and lower in calories have a higher nutrient density score. Among the advantageous nutrients in discussion are:

- Vitamins like A, C, K, D, B12, and E

- Minerals like potassium, magnesium, zinc, iron, and calcium.

- Protein

- Fiber

- Fatty acids like the omega-3s EPA and DHA

- Plant-based polyphenols and antioxidants

So if nutrient density was a university and fruits, vegetables, grains, and processed meals attended. Vegetables and fruits will always receive high scores; they would be the lecturer's favorites, whereas processed meals and grains will always get low scores. Some of you may be reading this and not see an issue with the traditional definition of nutrition density. But here is the thing: What this definition does is penalize calorie-dense whole foods like meat, fish, and avocados. These meals have high levels of fatty acids, protein, and micronutrients that are difficult to find elsewhere. To discourage you from consuming them is to invite nutrient deficits. Therefore, think about observing nutritional density and calorie density independently. Accumulating healthy nutrients should be the aim, not necessarily avoiding foods high in calories.

Getting Familiar With Bioavailability

A nutrient's bioavailability is the percentage of it that the body can use and store once it has been consumed. It is the percentage of a substance that is absorbed in the stomach and held in body tissue. Did you know that you cannot absorb the majority of the nutrients you eat? Also, did you know that the bioavailability of calcium from dairy is only 40%? Here is another fun fact: Kale has just 5% bioavailable vitamin K. However, I should point out that these are only approximations. Everybody is different; we are all structured differently, and therefore, each person will absorb a nutrient from a dietary source slightly differently.

Here are some factors that influence bioavailability:

- **The inclusion of additional nutrients**: For example, calcium absorbs more readily when combined with vitamin D.

- **The anti-nutrients existence**: For instance, phytic acid, also known as phytates, is a substance found in various things such as grains, legumes, nuts, and seeds that may prevent the absorption of minerals.

- **The nutritional form**: Heme iron found in meat, fish, and poultry, for instance, is more readily absorbed than non-heme iron that you get from plants.

- **Individual considerations**: For instance, people who have had gastric bypass surgery in the past or who have digestive problems may find it difficult to absorb vitamin B12 from food.

- **Preparing food**: Take for instance, cooked tomatoes, which tend to have a higher bioavailability rate and have the advantageous chemicals naringenin and chlorogenic acid compared to raw tomatoes. So you get more bioavailability when you cook them!

This is a lot to digest (no pun intended), but gaining this knowledge is beneficial in a variety of ways and will make you more mindful when you are making decisions in regard to food combinations.

How Do Antioxidants Impact Your Health?

Antioxidants are compounds that shield your body from the damaging effects of free radicals, which are unstable molecules. When electrons, which are charged particles, are added or removed from atoms in your body, free radicals emerge. Do not freak out; not all free radicals are harmful. They are crucial to numerous biological processes that your body needs, such as cell division. They also support communication between cells and aid in the body's defense against infection. Think of it like a WhatsApp group chat happening, and they send messages to help protect your body. Your body reads and follows instructions. Pretty cool, right? But here is the thing: An excess of free radicals can cause major harm to cells throughout the body. I am sure many of you were told growing up that too much of one thing is never a good thing. With an excess of free radicals in your body, diabetes, high blood pressure, heart disease, and cancer may all be exacerbated by this. In addition to being taken as supplements, antioxidants are naturally present in a wide variety of fruits, vegetables, and other foods. They can also be found in various skin-care items that many of you probably use. Antioxidants are often spoken about as a single category, but in reality, they belong to a large family. Antioxidants include beta-carotene, vitamin C, vitamin E, and vitamin A.

There are numerous others, each with its own unique advantages. Other antioxidants include:

- Glutathione

- Coenzyme Q10

- Lipoic acid

- Flavonoids

- Phenols

- Polyphenols

🌿 Phytoestrogens

However, a diet rich in fruits and vegetables is beneficial for numerous other reasons as well. Typical foods high in antioxidants are:

🌿 Tend to be dense in fiber

🌿 Tend to have low levels of cholesterol and saturated fat

🌿 They are brimming with nutrients and vitamins

🌿 Possess antioxidants to ward against cancer

Phytonutrients and Their Health Benefits

Phytonutrients play a huge role in your health and overall well-being. Plant foods like fruits, vegetables, whole grains, and legumes naturally contain phytonutrients. These plant-based compounds have very positive effects, and when they are combined with other necessary nutrients, they do wonders for your overall wellness.

The Breakdown

The word "phyto" means plant. The word placed together means plant nutrient. What I want to let you know is that there are many natural nutrients known as phytonutrients or phytochemicals. Carotenoids like lutein, flavonoids, coumarins, indoles, isoflavones, lignans, and plant sterols are essential nutrients found in plants. The amazing thing about phytonutrients is that they are potent antioxidants. As we get older, things change within our bodies, and the main goal that many of us try to achieve is to prevent deterioration. What if I told you that there are numerous phytonutrients that have antioxidant qualities that aid in preventing cell deterioration throughout the body? On my journey to health and wellness, when I learned this, it made me excited, and I hope it does the same for you.

Also, there is a barrage of phytonutrients that have been demonstrated to lower the risk of:

- Cancer

- Heart disease

- Stroke

- Alzheimer's

- Parkinson's disease.

I should also add that during my personal research, I came across studies that supported the belief that consuming meals high in phytonutrients in moderation encourages optimal aging. Phytonutrients have other impactful biological roles, such as:

- Enhancing your overall health

- There are some that are beneficial to your hormones and your immune system.

- They also contain antiviral and antibacterial properties.

List of Phytonutrient-Rich Foods

1. Tomatoes
2. Carrots
3. Peppers
4. Squash
5. Sweet potatoes
6. Peaches
7. Mangoes
8. Melons
9. Citrus fruits
10. Berries
11. Spinach
12. Kale
13. Bok choy
14. Broccoli
15. Swiss chard
16. Romaine lettuce
17. Garlic
18. Onions
19. Chives
20. Leeks

21. Brown rice

22. Wild rice

23. Quinoa

24. Barley

25. Wheat berries

26. Whole wheat

27. Whole grain breads

28. Whole grain cereals

29. Walnuts

30. Almonds

31. Sunflower

32. Sesame

33. Flax seeds

34. Dried beans, peas

35. Lentils

36. Soybeans

37. Soy products

38. Tea (specifically green tea, and black tea)

39. Coffee (black coffee)

40. Dark chocolate

To put it another way, the optimum diet for your health is one that consists mostly of plant foods that are high in phytonutrients. You should consume a healthy range of foods every day. There is no supplement that can match the advantages of eating a balanced diet. I am not knocking supplements, but going this route will always be my first choice, and I want it to be the same for you.

Chapter 2

Superfoods Are Your New Health Clique

Healthy eating is a way of life, so it's important to establish routines that are simple, realistically, and ultimately livable.

–Horace

Eat Right to Make Your Heartbeat Right

There are some foods that you can find easily that can lower your chance of developing heart disease. I am sure that when you read that, your heart probably leaped for joy. Your heart is so valuable to you that it should be safeguarded at all costs. It is only right that you look after your heart. You can lower your chance of developing heart disease by practicing mindful eating. These superfoods that are listed below are beneficial in aiding with the lowering of blood pressure, elevating good cholesterol levels, and also aiding in preventing plaque from accumulating in your arteries to protect your heart. They also contain fiber, potent antioxidants, beneficial fats, and vital vitamins and minerals.

The next time that you are preparing a meal, keep these superfoods in mind:

- **Dark leafy greens**: Dark leafy greens such as kale, spinach, and arugula are rich in nutrients, vitamins, and minerals. Especially an important B vitamin called folate, which is helpful for heart disease prevention.

- **Berries**: The flavonoids that are prevalent in blueberries, strawberries, goji, and acai berries are excellent choices from the superfoods list as they are extremely helpful with circulation by dilation of blood vessels and lowering blood pressure.

- **Olives and olive oil**: For years, olive oil has been known to have heart-healthy properties. Studies indicate that olive oil can lower blood pressure, triglycerides, and bad cholesterol levels while raising your heart health and fostering the rise of good cholesterol levels. If your life were being played out in a mystical movie, olive oil would be a potion people would be hunting for.

- **Fatty fish and fish oil**: The beauty of salmon, mackerel, and other fatty fish is that they are packed with omega-3 fatty acids. Omega-3 acids play an important role in maintaining a healthy heart. Now, I understand that there are many of you who may not be fans of seafood or even have an allergy. However, for those of you who do not have an allergy, consider purchasing fish oil to get the dose of omega-3 that your heart needs.

- **Beans and other legumes**: Beans and legumes are real due to their high content of plant protein, fiber, and other micronutrients, low-fat content, cholesterol-free status, and relatively low glycemic index. Beans and other legumes are extremely beneficial for cardiovascular health.

- **Mixed nuts and seeds**: We all, at some point, want a snack; however, sometimes we end up overindulging in unhealthy snacks, and there are some people who have limited control over snacks. This is where nuts and seeds are a great option and alternative. Nuts and seeds are great sources of not only protein but also healthy fat and other nutrients. Choosing unsalted nuts and making them a healthy snack alternative may reduce your risk of a heart attack.

- **Citrus fruits**: Citrus fruits have a variety of things in them that are good for your heart. Oranges, lemons, limes, tangerines, and kumquats are packed with vitamins and antioxidants.

🌾 **Whole grains**: I should let you know that consuming whole grains as opposed to refined ones will provide a better shield for your heart. Whole grains such as brown rice, buckwheat, oats, barley, quinoa, rye, and spelt are healthy and unprocessed.

Superfoods Are the Best Investment for Your Immune System

Although immunity is an important factor for 365 days of the year, over time, it seems to have gained even more attention as a health concern for many people. Also, let's be honest, it always piques our curiosity more during the winter—and maybe even the early spring. This is because that is when the dreaded cold and flu season arrives. All hope is not lost, as you may lower your risk of being sick and getting the sniffles by taking some simple steps to maintain and boost a strong immune system. Nutrition and sensible eating practices are two of the best methods to strengthen your immunity throughout your life. Also, make an effort to consume superfoods that are centered around strengthening your immune system. This will make it a bit more difficult to get a cold and if you do catch a cold or flu, you will find that your body will be able to fight off it quicker.

Listed below are a set of superfoods that are immune boosters:

🌾 **Leafy greens**: Yes, leafy greens are back on the list! As you learned above, leafy greens like kale, spinach, Swiss chard, and arugula are among the best superfoods to eat frequently since they not only boost brain and heart health but also cholesterol levels. Micronutrients found in leafy greens, particularly vitamin C and vitamin K, are abundant and extremely important for supporting a strong immune system. Leafy greens also contain pro-immunity elements like beta-carotene and folate, or vitamin B9. Try your best to shoot for at least two cups of leafy greens each day to ensure you're getting enough. Also, do not limit how you consume them, meaning that it does not have to be solely salads; there are more options: Try blending some greens into soups, stews, omelets, pasta dishes, and grain bowls, or try creating a tasty green smoothie. Mix it up!

- **Probiotic foods**: Probiotic foods like tempeh, yogurt, kefir, kimchi, and sauerkraut are some real MVPs when it comes to a healthy digestive tract. Additionally, because immunity and digestive tract wellness are connected, these probiotic-rich foods are multipurpose superfoods. How cool is that? Probiotic foods contain "good" bacteria that help the immune cells lining the intestines function better. These microbes also break down food so the body may absorb nutrients that would not otherwise be available. This guarantees your immune system receives the nourishment it requires to function at its peak. You should think about including probiotic foods in your food consumption at least two or three times a week for the best immune-supporting effects. Garnish your chicken tacos with sauerkraut, munch on naturally fermented pickles, or top your Greek yogurt with chopped nuts and berries in the morning.

- **Citrus fruits**: Vitamin C is key, and it is abundant in citrus fruits like grapefruit and oranges. Due to the fact that it stimulates the development of immune cells, or white blood cells, that fight disease, this vitamin is critical for optimal immunological function. You can eat citrus fruits by themselves, in fruit smoothies, or as a salad topping. Remember, variety is a great approach to a healthy life.

- **Berries**: When it comes to meals that strengthen the immune system, berries like raspberries, blueberries, and strawberries are a great choice. Remember in Chapter 1, I let you know the potent effects of antioxidants, which are abundant in berries? They are perfect for shielding healthy cells from harmful substances. Berries also give fiber, which supports the "good" bacteria in the digestive tract, and vitamin C, an important component for immunity (this is particularly found in strawberries). Aim for two half-cup servings of berries per week; this is simple to achieve with delectable dishes like smoothie bowls and berry-baked oatmeal. I mean, you could also just get them out of the refrigerator, wash them, and enjoy them. They are very tasty!

- **Lean Protein**: While plant-based superfoods are a good source of vitamins and antioxidants that support immune function, try not to forget that protein is equally important. Protein does, in fact, aid in your body's ability to create antibodies, heal muscles and tissues, and synthesize amino acids required for immune system function. However, when you are selecting proteins, always aim for lean proteins, as they are the healthiest choice because they contain less saturated fat.

- **Green tea**: I know many of you saw green tea and immediately rolled your eyes, but hear me out for a bit. It is actually possible to boost your immunity by sipping some green tea. A staple in any tea collection, green tea is incredibly earthy and refreshing. For some of you, after a while, it will become an acquired taste. Among the many antioxidants found in green tea is a plant material known as epigallocatechin gallate. This substance can help your body function better and lessen inflammation. Green tea can be consumed hot or cold; if this is still not that appealing to you, add it to a smoothie and see how you feel about it.

A Healthy Gut Is the Way to Keep Your Wellness Up

How our bodies are structured and designed is fascinating; everything in our bodies has a specific duty and plays a specific role. All our bodies are complex, multifaceted, and endowed with a wealth of amazing abilities. Despite all the other amazing aspects of our bodies, our digestive system is among the most vital organ systems that support all human beings. The digestive system of your body comprises the pancreas, liver, gallbladder, and gastrointestinal tract, which are responsible for breaking down the food and liquids you ingest throughout the day. Your body needs the nutrients, vitamins, proteins, and other ingredients in the foods and beverages you eat and drink to function correctly and be healthy. Everything is processed in your digestive system, which is why it is such an integral part of our bodies.

This is why it is imperative for us to eat the right foods, as it does wonders for maintaining a healthy digestive system. I will be listing superfoods and drinks that will help your digestive system:

- **Apples**: An apple a day keeps the doctor away. I believe almost all of us heard this growing up. This is not just a catchy line; apples are healthy, and they are good for you. We all love to snack, and not all the snacks we choose are healthy, and we also consume them in large portions. You should try taking as apple an alternative snack next time you feel hungry. Not only will it assist your digestive system and aid it in working more efficiently, but it will also provide you with enough energy to last until your next meal.

- **Avocados**: Many of you love spreading avocado on toast, and nothing is wrong with that, but avocado is not simply your go-to toast topping. In fact, it is packed full of potassium and fiber. If your digestive system could give you a high five for including it in your diet, it would.

- **Black beans**: Many people avoid black beans, but they are very beneficial to your digestive system. Oftentimes, we refuse a particular fruit or bean because of how we are used to it being prepared. This is where you all have to explore new recipes, and you may be shocked at how much you like black beans. Increasing your consumption of black beans is a great way to maintain a healthy digestive system. Not only do they maintain your digestive system, but they also give your intestines an abundance of beneficial microorganisms and help avoid constipation.

- **Ginger**: The spice that yields abundance! Ginger improves transit through your digestive tract and serves as a natural remedy for muscle aches and motion sickness. If your stomach is unsettled, ginger tea is a great remedy.

- **Leafy green vegetables**: Leafy greens are here again, guys! I did not want to say it, but I believe that leafy green vegetables are the MVP of superfoods. Rich in vitamins and nutrients, leafy green vegetables like kale and spinach promote a healthy digestive system.

- **Whole grain foods**: Whenever you are about to make or order a sandwich, you have the option to choose between white or wheat bread. Always choose wheat bread. For those of you who are rice lovers, make brown rice your rice of choice. See where I am going with this? Whole grains are a great source of minerals and fiber that your body requires for healthy digestion.

⚞ **Yogurt**: Do not make yogurt the item you skip in the supermarket because you feel it is the worst-tasting thing on the planet. However, to reap the digestive advantages that yogurt has to offer, you will have to consume it. There are many flavors out there that you can choose from, and I am sure you can find a flavor you like. Find new foods and drinks to stock your kitchen cupboards and refrigerator with that will keep your body in optimal condition.

Superfoods to Help You Kickstart Your Life

There are various superfoods that you can incorporate into your daily routine that can have amazing benefits for your joint health and help reduce inflammation. Joint pain and inflammation can be extremely uncomfortable, along with the fact that, in some cases, it limits how often you exercise and also limits what workouts you can do, which can be frustrating. I am not suggesting that you completely stop taking any prescribed medications from your doctor and swap them for superfoods. However, I have to let you know that there are superfoods that you can easily include in your everyday life that can greatly improve joint issues. If you experience joint discomfort due to injury or natural aging (we all have to face this), here are some superfoods that you should consider adding to your meal plan.

Although they will not cure arthritis or regenerate cartilage, they are all good for your overall well-being, and there is no harm in giving them a try.

Also, I would also suggest making notes to compare how your joints feel after incorporating these superfoods into your diet:

- **Fatty fish**: Omega-3 fatty acids, which are found in salmon, sardine, and mackerel, have anti-inflammatory qualities. Not only are these fatty fish tasty, but what is found in them can lessen stiffness and soreness in your joints. Not only do they have omega-3 fatty acids, but they also have the added bonus of vitamin D, which supports stronger bones. If possible, you should consume two servings or more each week.

- **Soy**: The beauty of soy is that it contains a lot of fiber and protein but little fat. Don't think I forgot about those of you who may not be fans of consuming fish because soy is a fantastic alternative and is high in omega-3 fatty acids, which enhance bone health.

- **Broccoli**: Do not leave out making broccoli a part of your life, as it contains sulforaphane, and sulforaphane may prevent the development of cells that result in rheumatoid arthritis.

- **Spinach**: Spinach is not only good for Popeye, but it has a load of benefits for your joints as it has a high concentration of antioxidants. What this does is reduce the effects of inflammatory agents and prevent the progression of osteoarthritis.

- **Walnuts**: I promote consuming healthy nuts and walnuts as one of them, and not only does it make a great healthy snack, but it has a barrage of health advantages. Nutrient-dense walnuts are great for improving joint health. They are high in omega-3 fatty acids and help reduce inflammation brought on by joint health.

- **Berries**: Not only are berries tasty, but they are also filled with nutrients. They are filled with a plethora of nutrients that can combat arthritis and can be found in berries like strawberries, blueberries, and blackberries.

- **Grapes**: Most of us love wine, and we appreciate grapes for that. But grapes offer more than just wine for us; the fruit includes substances like resveratrol and proanthocyanidin that improve joint health by lowering blood levels of inflammatory indicators.

- **Olive oil**: Olive oil has a variety of benefits; if you are consistent with taking it, it will lessen swelling in joints and degeneration of cartilage.

- **Cherries**: Cherries are not only a burst of flavor, but they also include anthocyanins, which are believed to have anti-inflammatory qualities and to lessen the incidence of attacks associated with gout.

🌿 **Ginger**: Ginger is packed with flavor; whether eaten fresh or dried, ginger reduces discomfort associated with arthritis.

🌿 **Garlic**: Garlic may not be the best-smelling or best-tasting when eaten raw. However, garlic has a reputation for lowering inflammation, and when consumed, it can lower your chances of developing hip osteoarthritis. Furthermore, it possesses cancer-fighting qualities and boosts immunity.

Chapter 3

The Superfood Prescription Plan

If you keep good food in your fridge, you will eat good food.

–Errick McAdams

You may be reading the information that I have presented so far and liking how it sounds. You would love to make it a part of your life, but you are not sure where to start. Well, I am here to let you know that it is not difficult to include superfoods in your diet.

Here are some basic tactics to get you going:

- **Smoothies**: Smoothies are tasty and are not complicated to make. The great thing is you can include what you want in it! There may be some

41

combinations that are not exciting to your taste buds, but you will find what works for you. and more importantly, you will be on a healthy journey. Make a healthy smoothie to start your morning off right by combining fruits, vegetables, and superfoods such as hemp, chia, and spirulina powder. Also, smoothies can be consumed for lunch as well. Mix and match various ingredients; trust me, you will find your ideal smoothie combo!

- **Salads**: Now, I know some of you saw the word salad and rolled your eyes. Salads do not have to be plain and bland. Thinking outside of the box is a great thing. Excite not only your eyes but your palate as well. For extra nourishment, add superfoods like quinoa, almonds, and mixed seeds; this will make your salad colorful as well as nutritious.

- **Oatmeal**: Oatmeal does not have to be prepared and placed in a bowl with no color. What you all should try, and do is add some crunch to your oatmeal by adding almonds, chia seeds, and flax seeds. Also, consider making your oatmeal more colorful and appealing by adding blueberries and bananas. Not only will it be healthy but filling as well, and you will have a hearty breakfast.

- **Yogurt parfaits**: Some of you are not fans of yogurt, but have you considered yogurt parfaits? Layering Greek yogurt, mixed berries, honey, coconut flakes, and pumpkin seeds results in delectable and nutrient-dense parfaits. This will be visually stimulating, and all those suggestions are healthy! The aim is to incorporate superfoods into your life and make the experience enjoyable as well. Healthy does not mean boring or plain.

- **Snacking**: Nothing is wrong with snacking; snacks are delicious! They are great to have when you are watching a movie or when you are relaxing with friends and family members. Now, yes, I love snacks, but I am team healthy snacks and I want you all to join the same team! Superfoods such as almonds, walnuts, pumpkin seeds, prunes, mulberries, and goji berries make for easy, wholesome snacks.

- **Baking**: For those of you who love to bake and try new baking recipes. Baking is a healthy option when not just preparing snacks but also when preparing certain meals. You cut back on oil use, etc. Incorporating superfoods like shredded coconut, almond flour, cashew flour, quinoa flour, and cacao powder are great options as they increase the nutritional content of what you are baking.

Quick Tips for Making Superfoods Part of Your Life

Now that you have options on how to start, what you want is for it to become a habit. The keys to retaining anything in your life are consistency and discipline. Or else you will do this for a week and revert back to old habits. To assist you in easily incorporating them into your everyday schedule, consider the following tips:

- **Take your time and start small**: What happens with many people is that they start big. Then, it becomes overwhelming, and they cannot maintain it. So, I advise that you start small and progressively add more superfoods to your meals, starting with one or two.

- **Make meal preparation a part of your life**: It is always a good idea to plan and prep; this way, you do not get overwhelmed and do not know what you plan on eating for the week. Therefore, for practical use throughout the week, wash, cut, and keep superfoods in easily accessible containers.

- **Nothing is wrong with experimenting**: Everything does not have to be exactly like what you see on a healthy cooking show or even what I share with you in my book. Nothing is wrong with taking the information gathered and placing your own twist on it. Examine a variety of superfoods to see which ones you prefer and how they might enhance your favorite recipes.

🌿 **Mix those flavors and watch how they excite your palate**: You will be shocked at how certain superfoods combined will excite your taste buds. Therefore, use inventive methods to blend savory and sweet superfoods to make your meals interesting and filling.

Overcoming Picky Eating and Food Preferences

I am sure most of you immediately saw a toddler or a child pushing away beans, lettuce, or broccoli. But there are also adults who struggle with eating those things as well. So what is a picky eater? The term "picky eating" describes a reluctance to try unfamiliar foods. It frequently goes hand in hand with a strong dietary preference. Foods with a particular taste or texture may be the focus of those preferences. For instance, a finicky eater could favor meals that are crunchy or simple to chew. There are some picky eaters who will only eat three specific things and nothing else, regardless of what nutritious aspects they may be lacking. On the other hand, some of you who are picky eaters could develop specific aversions to particular flavors, textures, scents, or even the appearance of food. Some adults and children who are picky eaters may avoid foods with green colors, creamy textures, or strong scents. The main issue with this is that you are robbing your body of things it needs. The truth is that it can lead to imbalanced eating patterns and inadequate nutrients. Studies show that picky eaters consume less meat, fish, fruit, and vegetables than average eaters. You will find that you have lower vitamin and mineral levels as well as iron and zinc, which may be a concern for certain finicky eaters.

Iron deficiency, especially in women, can lead to anemia and other illnesses.

So for those of you who are picky eaters and want to break free, here are some things that you can do:

- **Start small**: Introduce small changes to your diet. Do not overwhelm yourself and buy a barrage of new and exciting superfoods. Then you end up wasting it because you just cannot handle dealing with all this new stuff. Here is a fun fact for you: When big changes occur in tiny doses, your brain adjusts to them more readily. You will need to rewire your diet to accommodate your newfound taste and texture preferences. Try incorporating one new component into a single meal rather than organizing a week's worth of completely different meals, including strange foods (to you). Introduce a different meal that you used to dislike if, after a few days or weeks, you find that you like it more. Over time, your brain will form fresh neural pathways that will allow you to truly appreciate foods you never liked before.

- **Try new things at home first**: When making this change, try it in familiar territory, i.e., at your home. I would not advise you to go out with friends and/or family members and decide to embark on this new journey first. It will keep your mind at ease, and you will not be apprehensive about what they place in the ingredients or have to deal with feeling as if you are immature in front of your friends, etc. Remember to take baby steps.

🌿 **Take this time to combine what you like and what you do not like**: No, you did not read that wrong. When you take the time to add legumes, broccoli, etc., to something that you prefer and love, like for example, chicken wings. It would take at least three weeks of work to successfully get rid of past taste preferences. You could decide to add tomatoes to your favorite chicken sandwich. Or add more cheese to your spaghetti dish if you plan on adding more tomatoes to it. Whichever meal you already love and what you wish to start eating will determine what you choose to do.

🌿 **If you are not sure where to start, participate in a class**: You will find that you are more inclined to try and eat new foods in a classroom setting than when you make your first attempt at home. Your senses are pampered during the cooking process, and you become proud of the finished product. Try this method with the meals you detest most by enrolling in an online or local cooking class.

Your taste buds do not have to be the only factor in determining your favorite foods. Tips like the ones I have provided make it easy to overcome picky eating as an adult. Think about the things you want to start eating but don't particularly appreciate. You can reprogram your brain and expand your diet by experimenting with different approaches; there are a lot of wonderful dishes accessible for inquisitive cooks.

Misconceptions About Superfoods

Superfoods are undoubtedly loaded with health advantages; this is why I am for them, and I can attest to it. However, there are also a lot of myths and false beliefs about these nutrient-dense foods. These are some widespread misunderstandings and fallacies around superfoods:

- **All superfoods are costly and expensive**: This is a myth, guys! Don't get me wrong, there are some superfoods, like acai and goji berries, that can be pricey and more challenging to locate. However, there are many superfoods, like spinach, kale, and blueberries, that are easy to find and reasonably priced at your neighborhood grocery store.

- **Superfoods are the answer to every illness**: This is a big misconception. Now, while superfoods are a beneficial addition to any diet, they are not an all-encompassing remedy for all illnesses. The greatest strategies to be healthy are to have a balanced diet, exercise on a regular basis, and consult with your healthcare provider.

- **For superfoods to work, they must be ingested in large amounts**: This is not true. The key to a balanced life is doing things in moderation. The same rule applies to superfoods. Superfood consumption can be advantageous when done in moderation; please note that there is no need to overindulge. It is more crucial to eat a range of nutrient-rich foods than to consume high quantities of any one food.

- **Superfoods belong only to health enthusiasts**: This is not accurate. There are many of you who may have felt that this path is not for you because you are not a health enthusiast. Superfoods are beneficial for everyone to include in their diet! Regardless of your level of interest in wellness and health, superfoods are for you.

- **Superfoods are inherently nutritious**: Yes, superfoods are nutritious, but always keep in mind that they come in a variety of healthful forms, and always remember that they're not all made equal. There are some fruits that have natural sugar in them, and some are higher than others, which people with diabetes should not consume.

- **Superfoods do not cause any negative side effects**: This is not true. Superfoods are typically healthy for the majority of people who consume them, although some may have adverse consequences, such as stomach problems, after eating them. When adding new items to your diet, it is usually a good idea to start cautiously and observe how your body reacts. You may have allergies that you didn't know about; this is why I made sure to let you know that you should speak with your healthcare provider. Your wellness should always be the main priority.

I want you all to keep in mind that superfoods can undoubtedly be a beneficial addition to your diet and a great way of life, but it is crucial to dispel some prevalent myths and misconceptions about these nutrient-dense foods. Superfoods should not be ingested in huge amounts to have any benefits; they are not a solution for all illnesses. In addition, while certain processed foods may contain some elements from superfoods, they may also be heavy in harmful fats or added sugars. Superfoods are beneficial for everyone's day-to-day life and a great addition to a healthy way of life, but when adding new foods to your diet, it is imperative to monitor your body's reaction, start out slowly, and speak with a nutritionist, dietician, and/or your doctor.

Superfood to Consume at Different Stages of Your Life

What You Eat Will Fuel Your Life

Most teenagers need guidance on eating well. This is a young and carefree stage of their lives, and nutrition is not necessarily at the top of their list. It is essential that teenagers eat well because they are going through a time of tremendous growth and development. What a teenager consumes gives them the energy and nutrition they need to maintain their developing bodies and minds. All healthy foods have a place, but some superfoods offer that extra nutritional boost that developing teenagers require.

By receiving enough nutrition, they will, in return, gain maximum well-being, development, and efficiency at school and in sports by including these five superfoods in their meal plans on a regular basis:

- **Foods that have omega-3 fats**: A teenager's academic achievement and stress management are greatly aided by omega-3 fats, which are essential to brain growth and development. The main dietary sources of omega-3 fatty acids are found in eggs, walnuts, pumpkin seeds, and fish like salmon and sardines. Their bodies and minds will be grateful for this, and it will make eating healthy less challenging as they get older. It can be given to them as snacks, salads, or sandwiches on occasion. Try different recipes and ask them for their feedback; this is a great way to include them.

- **Consuming greens**: Most teenagers see greens, and they cringe and are immediately turned off. Among the most nutrient-dense foods are leafy greens. Which most teenagers are not the biggest fans of. However, it has few calories and a wealth of vitamins, minerals, fiber, and antioxidants. The best greens for them to consume are broccoli, asparagus, and lettuce. This is also where you are going to have to explore a variety of creative ways for them to actually consume these needed greens.

- **Blue is cool**: Colors in fruits and vegetables are a common theme. This is what makes them so amazing; they are not just all one color, but they come in a variety of hues, and they have unique flavors attached to them. Anthocyanins, which are often found in blue foods, help reduce oxidative stress in our bodies. This is great for teenagers as they go about their various challenges during this stage of their development. They contribute to their overall health and fight off free radicals that cause diseases. Common examples of blue foods are blueberries, blue spirulina, and damson plums, and they are filled with antioxidants.

- **Consuming red and orange foods**: Here come the colors again! Foods that come in this color group provide adequate amounts of fiber, potassium, and vitamins. You will find that this group comprises fruits like cherries and apples as well as vegetables like carrots, red peppers, sweet potatoes, and tomatoes.

- **Making whole grains a part of their regime**: Whole grains are rich in fiber, vitamins, iron, magnesium, and manganese. You can find this in buckwheat, whole wheat, and oats, which are a few types of whole grains. It can be a part of their breakfast meal and snacks, and it can reduce their risk of diabetes, heart disease, and weight gain.

Superfoods That Should Be a Part of Your Life During Your Menstrual Cycle

Many women find that their menstrual cycle is a very trying time due to hormonal problems, excruciating pains, and specific cravings for junk food or extremely sweet foods. Superfoods are ideal to eat during this time because they can be beneficial throughout this specific phase. Listed below are some superfoods that you should make a part of your routine during your monthly cycle.

- **Whole grains**: Whole grains are a great source of B-complex vitamins and vitamin E, and they are very beneficial to women during this time as they can assist with fatigue and mood changes. Also, when consumed an hour before going to bed, they can also help with PMS.

- **Pineapples**: Pineapples contain bromelain, which helps with reducing pain. I should also note that bromelain contains compounds that seem to decrease blood clotting and impede the formation of tumor cells.

- **Legumes**: Due to the fact that they are rich in Vitamin B, they are good for addressing all the various symptoms experienced by women during their menstrual cycle.

- **Yogurt**: Owing to its high calcium content, yogurt can be a great help for managing menstrual cramps and other related problems associated with menstruation.

- **Broccoli and kale**: Menstrual discomfort can be effectively relieved by consuming these two green superfoods, which are abundant in calcium, vitamins, and powerful antioxidants.

🌿 **Flaxseed oil**: Flaxseed is high in omega-3 fatty acids. This is a great option for women who are menstruating due to the fact that it forms prostaglandin, which reduces discomfort associated with the menstrual cycle.

The Best Superfoods to Eat When You Are Over 50

Many of you tend to be "stuck in our ways" after the age of fifty. There are things that have become a part of you that are hard to change or stop doing altogether. In fact, learning a new habit after it has been a part of your life for a year is challenging in and of itself. So after having something engraved in you for so many years, it can definitely be difficult to switch, but that does not mean it cannot be done. So, it could be that you have been a very healthy eater for the majority of your life. Or maybe you are someone who has not necessarily been a part of the healthy eating train. Regardless of which side of the wall you are on, making certain health and routine changes after fifty can be challenging. However, this is the time when you are going to have to be more careful with what you eat and also become a bit more picky. Not picky about not eating healthy food, but picky about the amount of alcohol you consume, ice cream, cake, and chips you eat. Whether it is casual or frequent, the truth is that our energy levels start to decline around middle age. That may be hard to read for some of you, but it is the truth.

Let us be honest. Around this time, you may notice that you do not have the room to drink as much as you used to or eat as many fries and cake slices as you did in your earlier years. Now, you start realizing that the weight is not dropping as quickly as it did, or in some cases, you gain weight way easier than you did before. No one likes or wants that; it fills you with a barrage of feelings and emotions. So, now you are faced with the reality that you may have to adjust to a slower metabolism, and that is just the tip of the iceberg. You also now have to deal with your bones weakening, changes in your bowel function, and a decline in muscle mass. There are a lot of things to process. I am not providing you with this information to make you run to the hills and scream but rather to make those of you in this age bracket more aware and make the necessary changes. When you are in this group, the best thing to do is to ensure that you are getting a lot of fruits, make it your point of duty to eat lean meats, such as chicken or fish (if you are still consuming meat), and put in the effort to ensure that you avoid saturated fats and sugars. Eating well and having balance in what goes into your body are great factors in reducing your probability of heart complications and are great ways of preventing you from getting diabetes, hypertension, and some cancers.

Listed below are superfoods that you must make a part of your life once you have hit the over-fifty mark:

- **Berries**: Berries are superfoods that anyone over fifty should ensure make it on their list. Berries contain fiber, and fiber does wonders for people over fifty, as it makes you go to the bathroom regularly and helps you keep your weight under control. And protects your body against diabetes and heart disease. Along with those wonderful elements, it contains vitamin C and has an anti-inflammatory agent. Berries are also wonderful for your brain as you get older, as they improve your motor skills and short-term memory.

- **Dark-green leafy vegetables**: As you get older, one thing will occur: Your bones tend to become softer, and calcium has to become your new best friend. You can get calcium naturally from dark-green leafy vegetables. Therefore, broccoli, spinach, kale, and arugula need to be on your shopping list when heading to the supermarket or market. They are also great for boosting muscle functions and your heart will love you for it as well, as they do wonders for keeping your heart healthy.

- **Seafood**: I am specifically referring to tuna, cod, and salmon. These tasty fish are a great source of protein. Fish is a wonderful source of B12.

- **Beans and legumes**: The great thing about beans and legumes is that they reduce cholesterol levels in your body. I don't know about you, but this is always a great thing to hear. They are also jam-packed with fiber and protein. You know that this is great for all body types, but this is an extra plus for those of us who are over fifty. It does not end there; they also contain iron, potassium, and magnesium. They are just filled with benefits for your body!

🌾 **Avocados**: Avocados are just filled with so many benefits! Let's be honest; they are also very tasty. But the thing I want to highlight is that they are great for your heart, and consuming avocados lowers your chances of cardiovascular disease significantly.

Chapter 4

100 Superfoods and Their Benefits

Let food be thy medicine, thy medicine shall be thy food.

–Hippocrates

There's a superfood? Yes, a superfood! Peeps, in this chapter, I will be listing 100 superfoods—yes, 100!. First, I will list them in categories and then look at them individually. Are you ready? Let's go!

Fruits	Avocados, Blueberries, Raspberries, Pomegranates, Strawberries, Blackberries, Cranberries, Cherries, Grapefruits, Apples, Pears, Kiwis, Bananas, Oranges, Mangoes, Watermelons, Acai, Goji, Pineapples,

	Rose Hip, Maqui Berry, Acerola Cherry, Lemon
Herbs	Turmeric, Ginger, Cinnamon, Garlic, Milk Thistle, Cacao, Black Pepper, Maca Root, Nutritional Yeast, Basil, Ashwagandha, Sea Salt, Rhodiola Rosea, CBD
Vegetables	Beets, Cauliflower, Asparagus, Broccoli, Sweet Potato, Tomato, Carrot, Kale, Eggplant, Snap Pea, Squash, Spinach, Celery, Cabbage, Cucumber, Collard Greens, Artichoke, Zucchini
Greens	Matcha Green Tea, Seaweed, Spirulina, Wheatgrass, Barley Grass, Chlorella, Moringa, Broccoli Sprouts
Proteins	Egg, Whey Protein Isolate, Collagen, Wild-Caught Fish, Grass-Fed Beef, Pastured Pork, Pastured Chicken, Bone Broth
Nuts, Seeds, & Legumes	Almonds, Chia Seeds, Flaxseed, Walnuts, Coconut, Macadamia Nuts, Chickpea, Pistachio, Beans, Lentils, Popcorn, Cashew, Pecan
Fats	MCT, Olive Oil, Avocado Oil, Ghee, Dark Chocolate
Mushrooms	Cordyceps, Lion's Mane, Chaga, Reishi
Digestive Support	Kefir, Sauerkraut, Kimchi, Inulin, Kombucha, Yogurt

1. **Acai berries**: These berries are packed with antioxidants, and they are good for your body and overall wellness. They also make great smoothies.

2. **Acerola cherries**: These cherries are filled with vitamin C. They are also good for your immune system, and they even have antimicrobial agents that can be very useful for skin blemishes and can even be used as a form of mouthwash. How cool is that?

3. **Almonds**: Almonds are not just the ideal little snack, but they are also quite healthy. They are rich in magnesium, which relieves blood pressure, controls blood sugar, eases muscle cramps, and even helps with sleeplessness. Additionally, it has a lot of vitamin E, which promotes overall skin health and wound healing.

4. **Apples**: This is not the forbidden fruit; do not run from them. Apples are great for your body. They have a lot of fiber, which is great for your digestive system. Having a great digestive system is a major plus!

5. **Artichoke**: This may not be at the top of your list of consume, but it does have a lot of benefits. Also, take some time and learn various recipes with artichoke; it does not have to be prepared one way. Artichokes are great for detoxification and digestion.

6. **Ashwagandha**: Ashwagandha, also known as white cherry, is grown in India. It is an adaptogen

that comes into great use during stressful situations. It also helps to promote brain function and is great for energy levels.

7. **Asparagus**: Asparagus gives your body a load of nutrition without adding a lot of calories. This should make you smile reading that, as I am about promoting health and a healthy weight. It is also full of antioxidants. These antioxidants include vitamins E and C, glutathione, flavonoids, polyphenols, and the flavonoids quercetin, isorhamnetin, and kaempferol.

8. **Avocado oil**: It is rich in monounsaturated fatty acids (MUFAs). This oil is great for reducing cholesterol levels. Eating avocados and using the oil that comes from them is a bonus! You can't lose.

9. **Avocados**: Monounsaturated fat is abundant in avocados. They are also high in fiber, minerals, including magnesium and potassium, and fat-soluble vitamins A and E. When consumed in conjunction with a nutritious diet, avocados may help reduce the risks associated with cardiovascular disease and control obesity.

10. **Bananas**: Bananas have a barrage of vitamins and minerals. But aside from that, this yummy fruit has two distinct carbohydrates. They are pectin and resistant starch; these two carbohydrates actually help to maintain your blood sugar levels. Soluble fibers like pectin help make your feces thicker, while resistant starch stays in your system for a

long period of time, and in doing so, it helps you feel full.

11. **Barley grass**: Barley grass is great for helping your body through detoxification. It also contains a healthy dose of vitamin C and is great for your immune system. Another great aspect of barley grass is that it really assists in alkalizing your body. If you want to aid with the digestive process, you should look into getting barley grass, as it is a good source of sodium, which is great for your tummy as it creates hydrochloric acid, which will be super beneficial in the digestion process. I should point out that you will most likely find barley grass in powder form. This is great to mix with water, and for those of you who are going to be all about smoothies, it is a great component to add, and it can serve as a good supplement.

12. **Basil**: Basil is categorized as an adaptogen. What this means is that it is an antioxidant that helps your body adjust to stress. This can be helpful for those of you who are in stressful jobs, as you will not become overpowered by stress. It also smells and tastes great, and it brings great flavor to your food.

13. **Beans**: Their rich and varied substance contributes to the development and upkeep of your bone structure. They assist in managing type 2 diabetes and are excellent for controlling blood sugar. They're also incredibly high in fiber! You need beans in your life.

14. **Beef**: Do you remember that "beef, it's what's for dinner" commercial? Well, beef is a great meal to include in your meals. I have to also highlight that the best kind of beef is one where the cows are fed grass. The beef from grass-fed cows is rich in omega-3 and richer in vitamins B and E, beta-carotene, iron, selenium, and zinc.

15. **Beets**: Similar to other foods with vibrant colors, beets are rich in anthocyanins, which are potent antioxidants. It is also relatively low in calories and will be great for weight loss; beets support heart health, enhance digestion, and even enhance brain function.

16. **Black pepper**: You are probably seeing this and wondering if I made an error. I am sure black pepper is the last thing you will expect to see on a superfood list. However, your blood sugar, cognitive function, and cardiovascular system can all benefit from those tiny black dots. I should point out that it might also facilitate the absorption of other beneficial elements, such as those in turmeric.

17. **Blackberries**: The great thing about superfoods is the variety of options, and you just cannot go wrong with berries. Vitamins C, K, and manganese are abundant in blackberries. Apart from micronutrients, studies have demonstrated that blackberry extract possesses potent antibacterial, antiviral, and anti-inflammatory characteristics in relation to oral hygiene treatments. Who doesn't want healthy teeth? I know I do! This is great

information to have. It is important to note that, in comparison to other fruits, they have a comparatively low sugar content (great news) and a high fiber content, which is also great news. Their low-glycemic status makes them an ideal choice for a nutritious snack and a great ingredient for smoothies.

18. **Blueberries**: Blueberries are not just tasty but are rich in nutrients; they are by far the most nutrient-dense type of superfood. Blueberries are an incredible source of micronutrients, including vitamin C, vitamin K, manganese, and antioxidants. They also have a high fiber content that is good for the digestive system. Specifically, berries and other red, purple, and blue foods have a vivid color because of antioxidants known as anthocyanins. It has been demonstrated that these substances are incredibly effective antioxidant scavengers and heart health guards.

19. **Bone broth**: Collagen is copious in bone broth; it will do wonders for joints as it promotes joint health. It will improve your digestion and make your skin look amazing. Bone broth is a good source of minerals since it is created by boiling bones for an extended period of time, breaking down the bone matrix. There are various bone broth recipes that you can find, and you can put your own spin on them so that your taste buds will do the happy dance.

20. **Broccoli sprouts**: Not many people talk about or venture into eating broccoli sprouts. So what exactly are broccoli sprouts? They are actually sprouted seeds of the broccoli plant. I hope you were not expecting me to go into a deep-rooted scientific explanation of what they were. They offer the same benefits as broccoli as well. If you are thinking of switching up your meal plan and adding something new and different, try broccoli sprouts.

21. **Broccoli**: Broccoli is good for your body! It has a lot of vitamin C, and it can be prepared in a variety of ways. This will allow your body to absorb not only vitamin C but also the antioxidants, vitamins, and minerals.

22. **Brussels sprouts**: They may be tiny, but they are jam-packed with vitamin K and antioxidants. I have to stress the importance of vitamin K, as it plays an important role in the healthy development of your bones and also helps keep osteoporosis from entering the chat room. Another important point I need to let you know about your new best friend, Brussels, is that they are high in fiber. Fiber is a key asset in assisting with healthy digestion and promoting a healthy tummy, and it is great for your cardiovascular health.

23. **Cabbage**: Cabbage is sometimes overlooked and underrated. It is a member of the Brassica family. Cabbage is nutritious and contains effective

antioxidants, vitamins, minerals, and glucosinolates.

24. **Cacao**: This is the main ingredient found in chocolate. Chocolate is one thing that most people love globally! Now, dark chocolate in moderation is beneficial to your health. But when you secure raw cacao, it has high levels of antioxidants. You can get it in its raw form (powder version) or in raw chocolate. Please remember that moderation is key.

25. **Carrots**: Carrots come in a variety of colors. They are not just orange! There are carrots that are white, yellow, red, burgundy, and purple. Carrots are rich in vitamins A and B. They are great for eye health; they are also rich in biotin, which is great for that skin glow; they are great for your hair, and they keep your nails healthy and strong.

26. **Cashews**: These nuts are high in fiber. They are also a great snack substitute for unhealthy snacks. They are good for maintaining healthy cholesterol levels and your blood pressure. They are also rich in copper and iron.

27. **Cauliflower**: Cauliflower is such a versatile vegetable that it can be prepared in a variety of ways to make healthier versions of common delights. You can either mash it to make low-carb mashed potatoes or shred it to make a low-carb pizza crust. Yes, low-carb pizza crust! It is tasty; I have prepared it myself! You may enjoy a creamy, dairy-free soup by blending some cauliflower with

a delectable bone broth. One of the few white foods abundant in nature, cauliflower offers a multitude of health advantages. One of its numerous advantages is that it contains glucosinolates, a sulfur component that strengthens the immune system against bacterial, viral, and fungal infections of the intestines and other parts of the body.

28. **CBD**: This is a non-psychoactive ingredient that is found in marijuana plants. It is legal and has received approval in the United States for both medicinal and commercial use. CBD has a beneficial effect on pain and inflammation by occupying the cannabinoid 2 (CB2) receptor.

29. **Celery**: Many restaurants serve buffalo wings (or any kind of wings) with celery. Due to its high-water content and crispy nature, celery is the perfect counterpart for the salt and fat that those tasty wings have. However, I am sure many of you push it to the side. You shouldn't, though. Here's why: Every aspect of the celery is edible and nutritious.

30. **Chaga mushrooms**: It is mostly sold as a tea or supplement and can be beneficial for cardiovascular health, blood sugar regulation, anti-aging, and inflammatory conditions like arthritis.

31. **Cherries**: Cherries have three amazing chemicals in them that have a variety of uses. They are tryptophan, serotonin, and melatonin. They have

different and important roles in your sleep and wake cycle. Melatonin plays a huge role in your falling asleep at night, whereas serotonin is the hormone that gives you a sense of well-being and high levels of content. Serotonin, which precedes melatonin, is derived from tryptophan. They are the power trio.

32. **Chia seeds**: Chia seeds are high in alpha-linolenic acid (ALA), an omega-3 fatty acid, and soluble fiber. In addition to their anti-inflammatory properties, the omega-3 fatty acids present in chia seeds have been shown to provide cardiovascular and mental health advantages. Diets high in fiber contribute to intestinal health and help regulate blood sugar. They contain a lot of protein, so don't let their size fool you.

33. **Chicken**: When purchasing chicken to consume, please ensure that it is pasteurized chicken. Most labels have a sticker letting you know that it is farm meat. Chicken meat from farms is loaded with vitamin D.

34. **Chickpeas**: Chickpeas are versatile and can be prepared in a variety of ways. They are very high in fiber. If you are a strict vegetarian or vegan, they will provide you with a high source of protein.

35. **Chlorella**: Chlorella is good at eliminating toxins and heavy metals, which is one of its primary medicinal advantages.

36. **Cinnamon**: Please do not attempt the cinnamon challenge. However, the ability of cinnamon to support normal blood sugar levels has led to an increase in its appeal among holistic health practitioners. But in terms of health advantages, it provides far more than that, such as anti-inflammatory and antioxidant aids for your body.

37. **Coconuts**: I have to make sure that I do not go on and on about coconuts. They are so good, guys! They have so many amazing qualities about them. Coconuts are super fatty (the good fatty that your body needs) and are lush in medium-chain triglycerides (MCT), which is a unique type of fat that aids in weight loss! And it powers your brain. Coconuts are also high in fiber, and you know what that means? Your colon will be very grateful and happy, and your digestive system will also be very appreciative. The water found in coconuts is rich in electrolytes, which are great for refreshing your body and giving you energy.

38. **Collagen**: In all our bodies, collagen is the most abundant protein. You may be aware that it is a component of connective tissue, skin, and nails. With a complete range of amino acids, collagen is a great source of animal-based protein that can help you gain and preserve muscle mass, which is great for your body. As you get older, it will be useful for keeping your skin tight and minimizing wrinkles. You can find collagen in most animal foods, but it tends to be more effective in bone broth. If you are

not into making bone broth or animal foods, you can purchase them in powder form; this may be more convenient for most of you. Having the powdered version of it will enable you to add it to your smoothies and coffee.

39. **Collard greens**: These leafy delights are popular in many Southern kitchens. They are packed with nutrients and very rich in vitamin K. Think about adding this to your list of items when you head to the market.

40. **Cordyceps mushrooms**: In China, there is a fungus called cordyceps that grows on the backs of particular species of caterpillars. Now that I know how that sounds, it may not be for everyone. But it supports healthy kidney, cardiovascular, sexual, and respiratory health. Additionally, cordyceps may support long life and a strong immune system.

41. **Cranberries**: Some of you only think about cranberries when it is Thanksgiving. Nothing is wrong with that. But I want you to have cranberries in your life more than just once a year, as they are great for your urinary tract. They are very low in sugar and high in antioxidants.

42. **Cucumbers**: Did you know that melons and squash are related? Well, if you didn't know, now you do. Cucumbers are filled with water (sounds similar to melons, right?) They are perfect for keeping you hydrated.

43. **Dark chocolate**: Dark chocolate is one of my favorite superfoods! I am going to let you know a little secret. Super dark chocolate is really viewed more as food than candy. So, I know that those of you who are watching your figure and want to stay healthy. Yes, it is tasty and great to eat. Now, all things must be done in moderation, so when you consume dark chocolate in moderation, you get more antioxidants in your body.

44. **Eggplants**: Eggplants can be prepared in different ways. There are various healthy seasonings that can be added to them, and they can be very enjoyable. You can find many recipes. Eggplants are very healthy, and they are also low in calories. Keeping the skin on adds to the nutrient level.

45. **Eggs**: Most of us love eggs; they are tasty. Not only are eggs tasty and can be prepared in a variety of ways, but they are also healthy fats and protein. Your yolks will be high in vitamins A and D if you ensure that you choose pastured eggs. Hens grown on pasture are free to move around, graze on their natural diet of grubs and seeds, and enjoy the sunshine. All of these contribute to the rich nutrients that can be found in eggs. While the yolk contains some protein as well as fat-soluble vitamins, the egg white contains the majority of the protein.

46. **Fish**: Fish (specifically wild fish) is a great source of protein. I made it a point to highlight wild fish because, unlike farm-raised fish, these fish eat

natural things. This will be beneficial to your body and will be filled with omega-3 fatty acids.

47. **Flaxseeds**: Flaxseeds have a lot in common with chia seeds, as they are also rich in fiber and the omega-3 fatty acid (ALA). Additionally, they contain a substance known as lignans, which has been shown to aid in the regulation of female hormones and reproduction. Though flax is more commonly used crushed than whole, just like chia seeds, it expands in water. I told you they had a lot in common. Here is a tip for you: Use flax meal as a vegan alternative to eggs in baking recipes, soak it in water, and let it swell.

48. **Garlic**: Not only great for warding off vampires (I couldn't help myself). Garlic is not only a tasty and aromatic addition to recipes, but it also contains potent antibacterial and immune-stimulating properties. Additionally, garlic has potent anti-inflammatory qualities.

49. **Ghee**: Ghee is mostly used in Indian cooking; however, ghee has gained popularity and appeal among paleo and ketogenic diet enthusiasts as a premium fat source devoid of allergies like lactose or casein.

50. **Ginger**: Ginger is a rhizome, and guess what? It is related to turmeric. Most of you know that ginger has the capacity to ease stomach aches. Several studies have shown that it can effectively help pregnant women with their morning sickness.

When taken in large quantities, ginger, a potent anti-inflammatory, has been demonstrated in studies to help lessen discomfort in the muscles. Its beneficial effects on blood sugar and cardiovascular risk factors—such as blood pressure and cholesterol level.

51. **Goji berries**: These berries have a bright red color. The color alone is appealing. However, they contain a strong source of zeaxanthin, which is known for its capability to protect your eyes. I know you are all for eye protection.

52. **Grapefruits**: I am not sure how many of you are familiar with the grapefruit diet. If you have, then you are aware of the great health benefits of grapefruit. Please note that I am not suggesting that any of you go on a grapefruit diet. Please remember that I am about balance, and I want that to be a part of your life. What I am highlighting is that there are many people who have tried that particular diet and discovered that grapefruits are packed with nutrients. What I will also highlight is that grapefruits are low in calories, have a low sugar level, and are also high in fiber. It is great to include it in your everyday eating, as it curbs your appetite (which helps with other eating) and enhances your health. Grapefruits are rich in a variety of nutrients that are great for your skin health and help fight infection. It contains zinc, copper, iron, and vitamin B.

53. **Inulin**: This particular powder is a fiber that can be found in various foods, like artichoke onions. It is regarded as a prebiotic food that supports the growth of good bacteria in your digestive system.

54. **Kale**: Kale is great for your body. Whether you choose to juice it or eat it raw, it does so many things for you. It is filled with micronutrients; it also contains beta-carotene and is rich in vitamins K and C.

55. **Kefir**: Kefir and yogurt have similarities, but kefir is packed with healthy bacteria. Yes, I said healthy bacteria. Don't freak out. It really is good for you. Kefir is a far more potent source of probiotics than yogurt, and this is due to the variety and abundance of microorganisms it contains. Although it is normally made with dairy milk, for those of you who are lactose intolerant, there are non-dairy versions of kefir that are just as rich in bacteria. There is even coconut water kefir. Kefir grains, collections of yeast and lactic acid bacteria, require a relatively short fermentation period (24 hours).

56. **Kimchi**: Kimchi is very similar to sauerkraut. It is a fermented cabbage and will provide your body with a barrage of nutrients. I should point out that this is a Korean staple. Kimchi is great for your immune health.

57. **Kiwi**: No, I am not talking about the Kiwi bird that represents the country of New Zealand. I am referring to this very delicious fruit that aids in

digestion and your overall digestive health. It also contains vitamins C, K, and E, folate, and potassium.

58. **Kombucha**: This beverage is sometimes referred to as mushroom tea. Various things can make this tea, such as black tea or green tea, lots of cane sugar, and a symbiotic culture of bacteria and yeast (SCOBY). It has probiotic benefits.

59. **Lemons**: They are not only great for making lemonades, but the citric acid contains health benefits. Now, you and I know that you cannot just grab a lemon and bite into it. But it can be added to certain meals because, when blended with other seasons, it makes the flavor pop. It can be added to water because citric acid has the ability to alkalize your body.

60. **Lentils**: Lentils are related to beans, all in the family. They are a type of legume. They are high in fiber, antioxidants, and minerals. They are great for cholesterol maintenance and minimize inflammation.

61. **Lion's mane mushrooms**: You must be wondering why I am flooding you with mushrooms at this point. Bear with me; it will all make sense. Lion's mane mushrooms are great for cognitive development. I am all about letting you know all the things that are great for a healthy brain.

62. **Maca root**: This Peruvian plant can be something you could consider for a smoothie (no, I do not

work for a smoothie company). However, smoothies are easy to prepare, they are healthy, and they should be something that you make a part of your diet. No need to worry; I will be including meal plans. Maca root can also be taken as a supplement. Studies done on maca roots show its potential to enhance the male and female libido. I should let you know that it has a strong nutty flavor; it is a bit of an acquired taste.

63. **Macadamia nuts**: Macadamia nuts contain a special type of monounsaturated fat (MUFA). This is good fat that you have seen me mention. They are high in fiber, and they make great snacks. They keep you full; this way, you will not feel the urge to keep snacking or overeating.

64. **Mangoes**: This is a tropical fruit, and most supermarkets have them. The common thing about mangoes is that they are very sweet, and they are delectable. They are very hard to resist and tend to be the top pick for many smoothies. Along with its tastiness, it has an abundance of vitamins and minerals, including magnesium and potassium. With these minerals present, it encourages healthy blood pressure and allows your blood vessels to remain calm. Maybe that is why I get this euphoric feeling when I consume them.

65. **Maqui Berries**: Also known as Chilean wineberry. They are small edible fruits that contain anthocyanins, which are great for your stomach and digestive system.

66. **Matcha green tea**: Matcha tea is a powdered version of green tea that is specially cultivated to support mental clarity and balanced energy. Who does not want higher mental clarity, support, and balanced energy? Compared to regular green tea, matcha has a higher concentration of an antioxidant called EGCG (epigallocatechin gallate).

67. **Medium-chain triglycerides (MCT)**: Fats derived from tropical plants, such as coconut and palm oil, include MCT fatty acids. For those of you following or interested in a ketogenic diet, MCTs can assist you in entering ketosis by increasing your metabolism and encouraging the synthesis of ketones. You purchase MCT oil powder and make it a part of your smoothie.

68. **Milk thistle**: This flowering plant is indigenous to the Mediterranean region. I should let you know that this is a superfood that you will find in pill, tincture, or tea form. This is due to the fact that it is really used mostly for medicinal purposes rather than culinary use. Your liver's natural detoxifying processes can be greatly supported and toned by milk thistle. It is not only beneficial for those suffering from cirrhosis but also for people with hepatitis or even type 2 diabetes.

69. **Moringa**: It is great for weight loss, and it contains anti-inflammatory properties. It is also great for reducing feelings of fatigue and enhancing your body's capacity to turn fat into energy.

70. **Nutritional yeast**: Nutritional yeast is a great addition to popcorn and eggs due to its flavor. For people who are vegans and vegetarians, this yeast is a great source of vitamin B and protein.

71. **Olive oil**: This oil is great to use to prepare meals as it is rich in monounsaturated fatty acids (MUFAs). Using this oil is great for reducing cholesterol levels.

72. **Oranges**: Most of us grew up being told that this citrus fruit is good for us as it prevents us from getting a cold. Now, it may not prevent you from getting a cold, but what it will do is make it a bit harder to catch a cold, and that is because it is packed with vitamin C.

73. **Pears**: This fruit is delicious and is a great addition to any fruit plate that you put together! This fruit is packed with fiber and antioxidants. It is also loaded with phenolic acids, which are known for their antimicrobial, anti-inflammatory, and anti-mutagenic aspects.

74. **Pecans**: Pecans have a very lovely taste. You cannot go wrong with it! It is high in fiber, it makes great snacks as it has a moderate protein level, and it contains a special kind of vitamin E called gamma-tocopherols.

75. **Pineapples**: Pineapples are so delectable! Many people still feel that it should never go on a pizza, while others think you are missing out if you have never tried a ham and pineapple pizza. One of the

many things we can all agree on is that it is a very sweet, and high-sugar fruit. Do not be alarmed; due to the fact that it contains fiber, it creates an even balance. It also has a high amount of vitamin C and manganese. Vitamin C is a great boost for your immune system, and manganese is great for your metabolism.

76. **Pistachio**: This is one of my guilty pleasures. They are very delicious, and not only are they delicious, but they are encumbered with nutrients! The green nuts are fun to look at and tasty, but they are great sources of lutein and zeaxanthin; these two nutrients are important for your eye's well-being.

77. **Pomegranate**: Superfoods like this one are tasty and are also nourishing treats that are loaded with fiber, vitamin C, vitamin K, and folate. This tangy, sweet fruit has antioxidant and anti-inflammatory properties that support a healthy digestive system.

78. **Popcorn**: No, this is not on the list by mistake. Popcorn is, in fact, a healthy food; it contains polyphenols, which have been linked to improved blood circulation and digestion. It is also a low-calorie snack. Here is the thing, though: The type of popcorn you will have to purchase is not the one you place in the microwave. You will need an air popper.

79. **Pork**: Pasteurized pigs are also the type of pigs that your pork should come from if you are a meat lover. Remember that pigs are omnivores by nature; they

don't need to limit their diet to just grass. However, the manner in which conventional pigs are treated is appalling from a humanitarian standpoint. They live in cramped indoor cages called concentrated animal feeding operations (CAFOs), which are riddled with disease and excessive waste. It puts the animals through excessive stress, and the stress hormones find their way into the meat you eat. The last thing you need to consume is meat packed with stress hormones. This is why you must ensure that you make sure that the meat you purchase is pasteurized. Pastured pigs have the freedom to roam the field and get healthy amounts of sun, which provides a huge boost to the meat you consume.

80. **Raspberries**: In addition to having minimal sugar content, raspberries are high in fiber, vitamin C, and manganese. They go well with salads, smoothies, or even just as a late-night snack.

81. **Reishi mushrooms**: These mushrooms are especially great for boosting your immune system and reducing inflammation. These are great to add to meals; they are not only tasty but also have great health benefits.

82. **Rhodiola rosea**: You may or may not be familiar with this herb. However, it is mostly enjoyed as a tea for some and a dietary supplement for others. It is great for calming your body and dealing with stress.

83. **Rose hip**: This is pseudo-fruit; it is not something that you typically consume, and it is rather done in tea form. It contains anti-aging agents, promotes the production of collagen, and has a high level of vitamin C.

84. **Sauerkraut**: Just like kefir, it is rich in healthy bacteria. What sauerkraut is lacto-fermented cabbage, but when you are purchasing it, please ensure you look for the ones labeled "raw"; otherwise, you probably will not get the healthy bacteria you want. Consuming a variety of meals high in healthy bacteria will strengthen your immune system and maintain the biodiversity of your gut flora. It is also strong in fiber and filled with vitamins K, C, and A.

85. **Sea salt**: You may be wondering what the difference between table salt and sea salt is. Well, sea salt has way more minerals than table salt. Table salt is merely sodium chloride. Meanwhile, sea salt has calcium, potassium, magnesium, iron, and molybdenum.

86. **Seaweed**: I know there are some of you for whom the word alone made you go "no!" However, hear me out for a second. Although seaweed is sometimes referred to as "sea vegetables," it is really an alga. Also, they do not come in one color; in fact, sea vegetables come in a variety of forms and colors, such as red, green, brown, or black. They are all high in tyrosine and iodine, which have different advantages. The standard American diet

(SAD) severely lacks these two nutrients, which are vital to thyroid health. Here is an unknown fact: the omega-3s found in fatty fish are derived from seaweed. For vegetarians and vegans who wish to increase their omega-3 intake without consuming fish, this is wonderful news.

87. **Snap pea**: Snap peas have less starch than regular garden peas, but they are still a bit sweet. They are high in fiber and contain vitamin C.

88. **Spinach**: Did you know that spinach is related to quinoa and beets? Spinach contains roughage, which is good for healthy and frequent bowel movements. It also has vitamins A and B9 (folic acid). Folic acid is very beneficial for pregnant women and mothers who are nursing.

89. **Spirulina**: Spirulina, which is sometimes referred to as blue-green alga, is a single-celled organism. It is one of the most nutrient-rich foods on the planet (yes, I said the planet). Due to its abundance of beta-carotene and other antioxidants, there is now research being done on it and how it affects allergies and cardiovascular health.

90. **Squash**: There are a variety of squash; to be honest, they should have their own slot on the massive list. However, I am going to be focusing on their textures. Winter squash (like pumpkins, butternut, spaghetti, and acorn) is very firm, and it cannot be consumed raw. They have a higher starch content than summer squash. Summer squash is softer and

more delicate (like yellow squash and zucchini); it has a thinner skin, and the flesh is more watery. Summer squash is lower in carbs compared to winter squash. However, the one with the lowest carbohydrate level is winter squash.

91. **Strawberries**: I may have a slight bias toward the Berry family, but can you blame me? Strawberries are packed with fiber and have a low sugar content. This makes them a great snack or dessert if you are trying to shed some weight or maintain your current weight.

92. **Sweet potatoes**: Sweet potatoes are packed with nutrients and fiber. But guess where that is located? In the skin of the sweet potatoes, it is a reflex for most people to peel the skin of potatoes, fruits, etc. However, I urge you to leave the skin on when preparing sweet potatoes to get all the benefits they have to offer. They are also filled with vitamins, minerals, and antioxidants. They come in different skin tones: orange with brown skin, white with red skin, and purple with purple skin. While each of them has a unique antioxidant aspect, there are some commonalities with other micronutrients such as potassium, manganese, vitamin B6, vitamin C, and vitamin A (in the form of beta-carotene).

93. **Tomatoes**: Lycopene-rich foods are rare on Earth; lucky for us, we have access to tomatoes as they are packed with lycopene. Lycopene is a carotenoid that is found in the skins of the tomatoes. Due to the fact that tomatoes come in so many varieties

and hues, their nutrient profiles vary slightly, but lycopene is always present. I have to highlight that the more red a tomato is, the higher its lycopene content.

94. **Turmeric**: Turmeric has entered the chatroom! Curry gets its golden color from the turmeric. There is a potent antioxidant called curcumin that is abundant in turmeric. Whether it's in a tea, a recipe, or a pill, you can ingest turmeric on a daily basis. By doing this, you may be contributing to a healthy detoxification process in your body and preventing inflammation. It also does wonders for your skin and helps to minimize dark spots.

95. **Walnuts**: Walnuts are another incredible nut that provides a wealth of antioxidants and a fantastic dose of fiber. They are a superb plant-based supply of anti-inflammatory omega-3s. Over time, it has been demonstrated that these delicious nuts can help with hunger suppression, weight loss, and willpower in relation to unhealthy foods.

96. **Watermelons**: I call watermelons the water fruit. This is because this fruit is 92% water-based. How great is that? It is great to consume during the summer, as it keeps you hydrated. They also contain a lot of lycopene, which is an important component for good eye health.

97. **Wheatgrass**: Most people tend to link wheatgrass with a great cure for an awful hangover. But it can

do more than that; it also has great anti-inflammatory properties.

98. **Whey protein isolate**: This protein is easy to digest and absorb into your system. The great thing about this is that it is ideal for those of you who can only tolerate minimal quantities of dairy products. It is the complete package; it is almost like a super protein as it contains all nine of the essential amino acids. Let that sink in for a minute! It also includes very important non-essential amino acids such as aspartate, arginine, and cysteine are also present. These amino acids are crucial for insulin production and aid in the growth of muscle mass. If you are working out with weights, this is a great superfood that you should add.

99. **Yogurt**: Probiotics are abundant in yogurt and other fermented foods. Probiotics are good microorganisms that reside in your digestive system.

100. **Zucchini**: Zucchini has a high water content and also has a high level of fiber. All parts of zucchini can be eaten. It has excellent effects on your thyroid, a healthy prostate, and strong bones.

Chapter "Good Will"

Helping others without expectation of anything in return has been proven to lead to increased happiness and satisfaction in life.

I would love to give you the chance to experience that same feeling during your reading or listening experience today...

All it takes is a few moments of your time to answer one simple question:

If so, I have a small request for you.

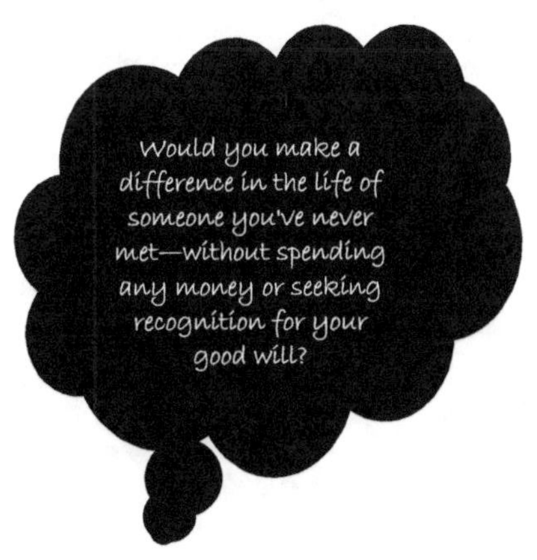

If you've found value in your reading or listening experience today, I humbly ask that you take a brief moment right now to leave an honest review of this book. It won't cost you anything but 30 seconds of your time—just a few seconds to share your thoughts with others.

Your voice can go a long way in helping someone else find the same inspiration and knowledge that you have.

Are you familiar with leaving a review for an Audible, Kindle, or e-reader book? If so, it's simple:

If you're on **Audible**: just hit the three dots in the top right of your device, click rate & review, then leave a few sentences about the book along with your star rating.

If you're reading on **Kindle** or an e-reader, simply scroll to the last page of the book and swipe up—the review should prompt from there.

If you're on a **Paperback** or any other physical format of this book, you can find the book page on Amazon (or wherever you bought this) and leave your review right there.

Chapter 5

The Pros and Cons of Superfood Supplements

Any food that requires enhancing by the use of chemical substances should in no way be considered a food.

–**John H. Tobe**

How to Evaluate Superfood Supplements

How can you truly assess a superfood supplement's reliability and efficacy or whether it lives up to all its claims? You want to make sure that the decision you make is best for your body and not something that really serves no purpose. The harsh reality is that it can be a bit tricky, and in some cases, depending on the supplement, it is not an easy task. Supplements, whether they are pills, liquids, or powders, are not subject to the same level of examination as drugs and are considered more like food than pharmaceuticals. This is something that not many people are aware of. In fact, according to the Dietary Supplement Health and Education Act that was passed in 1994, the majority of substances in supplements were categorized as generally recognized as safe (GRAS) and are considered safe unless there are adverse impact reports that provide evidence to the contrary. The Food and Drug Administration (FDA) must be informed about and given proof that a supplement is reasonably believed to be safe before a company can offer a new supplement or dietary ingredient. Therefore, it is a very good idea to discuss any concerns you have about a supplement with your healthcare provider and conduct your own independent research to look into claims, interactions with other medications, and possible negative effects.

When selecting a supplement, I also suggest that you take your time and read the label carefully to make sure the dose recommendations, claims, and warnings are clear and concise. When describing how a supplement may impact your body's structure and function—rather than a specific illness or medical condition—suppliers typically make what are known as "structure-function" claims. They usually include a disclaimer stating that the FDA has not reviewed the claim and that the product is not meant to diagnose, treat, cure, or prevent any disease. They tend to also frequently use terms like "promote," "benefits," or "maintains." I advise you to seek reliable, fact-checked websites where you may learn more about the supplement and/or supplements you are thinking about purchasing and consuming and ask questions regarding its efficacy, interactions with other medications, restrictions, and adverse effects. Even though they may be claiming to be superfood supplements, I want you all to choose wisely and make accurate decisions. Also, ensure that you check for supplements that are packed with added flavors and check the sugar content. Your basis should be focused on what the superfood supplement has to offer more than the taste.

Potential Risks and Other Things to Consider When Purchasing Superfood Supplements

Superfood supplements serve many purposes; these powders are very common and are used by many people, and this will be my main focus. Superfood powders are made from entire foods that have been dried and processed into a powder. A combination of multiple dried whole meals or a single food can be combined to create a superfood supplement powder. You have the option of purchasing them in health food stores or online, and if you choose, you can watch tutorials online and make them yourself. They can be added to liquids that will make them easier to drink, and/or you can add them to whatever meal you are consuming to boost their nutritional value. Superfood powder contains a high level of nutrients, including proteins, vitamins, minerals, and enzymes. Most of the powders are often green in color because they contain plants that are lush in chlorophyll. If you locate a super green superfood powder, it tends to be a blend of spinach, broccoli, wheatgrass, alfalfa sprouts, green cabbage, kelp, basil, asparagus, barley grass, and spirulina.

I have to be fair and not only list the many benefits but also list the cons associated with them.

This will give you a great level of insight and assist you in deciding which is the best superfood powder supplement for you.

The Benefits of Superfood Powder

- **They are quick and easy to make**: Many of you live a pretty fast-paced life, and every second counts. Superfood powders take a minute or two at most to mix and make a drink that you can take with you as you head to work or before going to the gym. For you to consume the same amount of nutrients, it would take longer if you were to prepare a meal.

- **There will be no wasted food**: Let's face it, sometimes the fruit and vegetables you purchase end up being spoiled or wasted. Also, fresh fruits and vegetables need to be eaten within a few days, as the longer they sit, their nutritional value starts to drop. Sometimes, you unintentionally forget about your produce. However, the great thing about this supplement is that it has a much longer shelf life than the fruits and vegetables you purchase. What this means is that you will not end up throwing away packets of your superfood powder on a weekly basis.

- **You will save a lot of fridge space**: Eating superfoods means that you will need quite a bit of whole foods. While I am all for you getting this, I am also aware that not everyone has a fridge size that can accommodate all these items. Superfood powders do not take up that much space and will make it easier for you to store them and not rob your body of the nutrients that you need.

- **It gives you a creative way to place nutrients in food**: There are some children and adults who are very picky eaters and do not like vegetables or fruits. They find it hard to consume them. Also, you do not want to rob your body or your children's body of the nutrients it needs. Blending these powders in sauces, yogurts, smoothies, and porridges is a great way to provide you and everyone in your family with the necessary nutrients.

- **It can give your immune system a great boost**: There are many superfoods that are great immune boosters; they will help fight off viruses and aid recovery from colds, etc. There are superfood powders that offer this, and there are supplements that contain broccoli or turmeric that could offer immune health benefits.

The Downside of Superfood Powders

While there are many benefits, there are also some downsides:

- **You may end up relying too much on supplements**: Let me be clear: There is no supplement (powder, pill, etc.) that will outweigh having a healthy and balanced diet. Most people tend to gravitate towards getting these supplements because they feel it gives them a pass to eat poorly and that their supplement will make up for it. To be frank, taking supplements alone will not give you all the amazing benefits that a healthy and balanced food diet will. When I say the word diet, I am referring to a lifestyle change, as this should not be temporary but an ongoing thing. Also, if you manage to eat right and eat an array of fruits and vegetables in a variety of hues, you will get all the nutrition you need.

- **They are expensive**: Listen, superfood powders are pricey. It requires a lot of ingredients to make a tiny portion of these dried powders. It is actually more cost-efficient if you make them yourself (and even so, it is still costly), but it is better to just get the fruits and vegetables at the market.

- **You may not really get what you paid for**: Not all superfoods keep it natural and pure. There are some superfoods out there that are not made from good-quality whole foods. Instead, they are filled with a barrage of chemicals and flavors. So that they are tastier, and people will gravitate towards them, but they serve no real purpose nutrition-wise to your body.

- **You will lose a sense of enjoyment with regard to eating**: Consuming these powders will make your whole "eating" experience bland and routine. Superfood powders are not nearly as delectable as a fruit bowl with a mix of berries, oranges, and apples. Or avocado on your toast.

🌿 **Taste-wise, they are not really that appealing**: Not many people like how these supplements taste. There are some of these supplements that have a real acquired taste; you may find yourself gulping them down just to be done with the experience.

Popular Superfood Supplements and Their Benefits

It is best to practice eating superfoods (organically); they have great benefits, as I have highlighted. However, I am aware that, based on various factors in your life, it may not be possible to consume superfoods every single day. This does not mean that you cannot still access the benefits of superfoods. You can look into purchasing superfoods in the form of supplements. I will be looking at superfood supplements in powder form. Superfood powders are frequently made by grinding up dehydrated whole foods, such as fruits and vegetables, herbs, or other botanicals, and then adding them to a variety of food styles, smoothies, and other recipes. Superfoods, such as berries and leafy greens, are renowned for their nutrient-dense qualities, which can help to strengthen your immune system, increase your natural energy levels, and give your body essential antioxidants. Additionally beneficial to digestion and general gastrointestinal (GI) health are superfood blends containing multifunctional fibers along with additional components. Superfood powders are becoming more and more popular, but not all of them live up to the same expectations. I have made a list of a few of the most popular superfood supplement powders, along with their pros and cons.

Superfood Supplement	Pros	Cons
Organic veggies	It contains 31 powerhouse ingredients (including dark leafy green, root vegetables, berries, and herbal botanicals) Great for your digestive system as it contains digestive enzymes Probiotics	This supplement can be a bit pricey. It has an earthy taste to it, which may not be favored by many.
Moringa powder	It is sustainable Contains antioxidants and anti-inflammatory properties	It has a very strong veggie flavor. (Acquired taste) Single superfood
Organic superfoods powder	Plant-based (contains buckwheat, quinoa, etc.) Fiber-rich (garbanzo beans, lentils)	It is not a significant source of fiber. Depending on the brand you purchase, there may be a high level of flavor added.

	Nutrient-dense (pumpkin, sunflower, and chia seeds)	That will rob it of its nutrients
Beet powder	Promotes blood flow Good source of iron	Depending on the brand (especially if it is flavored, there will be high levels of flavor that will rob it of its nutrients) Single superfood
Maca root powder	Rich in fiber and vitamin C Easy to blend No preservatives or artificial ingredients	Single superfood The sustainability of Peruvian maca is unsure
Mushroom powder	Contains plant adaptogens	Has a strong flavor Not for blending with other foods
Cacao powder	Increases blood flow to the brain	Limited uses
Lucuma powder	Sweetener alternative Vitamin C Great for smoothies	Limited uses
Acai powder	Contains omega-6 and omega-9 fats	Single superfood

	Has a sweet berry taste	
Goji powder	It is a good source of vitamin A, selenium, and copper	Single superfood
	Has antioxidant	

Chapter 6

Overcoming Challenges

Self-care is not selfish. You cannot serve from an empty vessel.

–Eleanor Brown

Budget and Accessibility Issues of Superfoods

There are many of you who do not feel that the path of wellness is not for you due to the fact that you think that in order to maintain and keep up that lifestyle, it will burn a hole in your pocket. To be honest, there are some superfoods that are more expensive than others, and various things affect whether you can get certain things. It could be your location, or it could be that your budget is super tight because you have a huge family. However, all hope is not lost, as I will help dismiss the claim that eating healthy will leave you healthy but make you broke. I will list items that you can store in your kitchen that will be essential and great for you but will not leave you looking for coins under the carpet to help foot the bill:

- **Rice and beans**: Beans and rice make a great combination. Not only are they healthy, but they are inexpensive and a rich source of nutrients, including fiber and protein. Discover how to harness their versatility to prepare satisfying meals that won't put your health or budget in jeopardy.

- **Oatmeal does not have to be only a breakfast meal**: Oats are a great superfood that is very affordable. At the same time, many of you may prefer it as a breakfast meal. It can actually be consumed for lunch or dinner. You can think outside the box about meals and not label everything one way and one way alone.

- Despite what you may think, **leafy greens** are not going to burn a hole in your wallet or purse. There are many leafy-green options that I have listed for you. Go through the list and find the ones that are within your price range.

What About Proteins?

Protein is an essential component of a healthy diet, and luckily, there are affordable options available. I will help you select protein sources that are both affordable and high in nutritional value.

- **Eggs**: This protein-rich food source will not make you scream at the cash register. You can prepare different meals with eggs because they are versatile.

- **Meats**: You should take the time to take a look at low-cost meat cuts that are pasteurized and will still give you the nutritional value that is essential to your body.

- **Plant-based options**: There are many plant-based foods that are packed with protein for people who are not into meat or eggs. Now, depending on where you live, the prices vary. However, it is not impossible to locate vegan meat, cheese, etc. You will have to do your research, compare prices, and decide which location is best for you. It can be done, guys.

Healthy Snacks on a Tight Budget and Smart Shopping Tactics

We all like a nice snack to have when watching a movie or if you had dinner very early and just feel for a snack afterwards. This is still achievable on a budget and will not compromise your wellness goals. When shopping, look out for reasonable, satisfying, and nutrient-dense snacks like popcorn, nuts, fruits, and seeds. They will satisfy your snack cravings without costing too much. You see that you can still snack, and there are various recipes that you can look up online that will assist you in making your own snacks. Sometimes, you already have the ingredients in your home and may not have considered making them into your own snacks.

Aside from snacking, here are some good shopping tactics that you should consider:

- **Consider shopping in bulk for certain items**: This actually lowers waste and saves money. Take the time to discover how to stock up on supplies without going over budget when it comes to shopping for your kitchen.

- **Discounts, sales, and coupons**: There are times that some people overlook this and miss out on deals to save money when shopping. Nothing is wrong with using this method. The world of promotions and deals is easy to navigate. Learn where and when to find the best prices so you can shop healthily without going over budget.

- **Organizing meals to save money**: It is time to tap into the possibilities of cooking. Meal planning allows you to reduce food waste and save money. Do not worry; I have included meal plans in the appendix section of my book.

Remember that achieving health and wellness is an ongoing journey; it is not a race. Take your time and be patient with yourself. If you approach your health goals with a balanced attitude, you can achieve your health goals while still being financially secure. Always remember to set realistic goals. When you embark on this new life-changing adventure, reconsider how you feel about eating healthily. You will discover that, with the help of inexpensive superfoods and wise purchasing strategies, achieving and maintaining wellness is feasible on any budget. Get ready to welcome a more contented and well-being version of yourself. Congratulations!

Superfoods That Can Help With Diabetes and Blood Sugar Management

For those of you who are reading my book and are dealing with diabetes, you are aware that you have to be conscious of the foods you consume, as they may influence your blood glucose level. As part of a balanced diet, some foods can assist in controlling your blood sugar levels. Damage to your blood vessels and nerve cells may arise from persistently elevated blood sugar levels. This can harm every organ in your body, including your kidneys and eyes, and will increase your risk of developing diseases and getting a stroke. Having a good diet is one strategy to control your high blood sugar. Eating a healthy diet can help prevent type 2 diabetes and avoid the worsening of diabetes's symptoms and effects. I will be listing superfoods that will be beneficial to those of you who have diabetes. These superfoods will also help you manage your blood sugar levels.

Please note that I am not encouraging you to stop taking your medications. What I will be providing are superfoods that you should consider becoming a part of your day-to-day life. You and your body will love what these superfoods may do for you:

- 🌿 **Avocado**: Avocados provide a good supply of healthy fat and roughly 20 different vitamins and minerals. Potassium, lutein, beta-carotene, and vitamins C, E, and K are also very abundant in avocados. Remember that consuming foods high in good fats contributes to your feeling full and prevents you from overeating. You may be wondering what that has to do with diabetes. Well, consuming fat slows down how quickly carbs are absorbed, which promotes more stable blood sugar levels. Also, avocados are very high in fiber. Researchers have found a strong correlation between a high-fiber diet and a markedly decreased risk of diabetes and its various complications. Evidence of the potential benefit of vitamin E supplementation for oxidative stress and glucose regulation in overweight people with diabetes was discovered in research conducted in 2004. (Manning, 2004)

- 🌿 **Chia seeds**: Chia seeds are loaded with fiber, magnesium, omega-3 fatty acids, and antioxidants. For those of you who have been told by your doctor to start monitoring how you eat as you are at risk of developing type 2 diabetes, each of these could lessen the chance of developing type 2 diabetes and its associated issues.

- 🌿 **Ginger**: Anti-inflammatory foods are sometimes defined as plant-based foods that are filled with antioxidants. This is due to the fact that they have the ability to reduce inflammation; they may aid in the treatment of symptoms as well as minimize the long-term risks of conditions like diabetes. Ginger's high antioxidant content suggests that it may have anti-inflammatory qualities.

- **Pumpkin seeds**: Pumpkin seeds are rich in fiber, magnesium, and good fats. Magnesium is necessary for more than three hundred bodily functions; yes, I said three hundred bodily functions, including the metabolism of food into energy. The polymers that are included in pumpkin seeds could aid in blood sugar regulation, which is something that those of you who suffer from diabetes need. Diabetes is one of the main causes of low magnesium levels in those with insulin resistance.

- **Spinach**: When you consume low levels of potassium, it increases your risk of diabetes and the various complications that come with it. Spinach contains a great source of dietary potassium, so it should be included in your meals.

- **Strawberries**: You already know that I am a big fan of berries! If you are not a fan, I am trying to make you join the team. Yes, they are tasty and easy to consume, but they are also a wonderful source of antioxidants. There was research that was conducted in 2011 that discovered that fisetin, which is derived from strawberries, shielded diabetic mice's kidneys and brains from damage. (Maher, 2011).

- **Tomatoes**: Tomatoes also have some MVP status on this list as well. The glycemic index (GI) of fresh, whole tomatoes is low. You may be wondering why I needed to highlight this. Well, low-GI foods release sugar into your bloodstream more gradually and are less likely to cause a surge in blood sugar levels. One reason for this being a factor with tomatoes is also due to the fact that they also supply your body with fiber. Keep this fun fact in the back of your mind. You may feel fuller for longer thanks to these two reasons. Consuming tomatoes may also lower the cardiovascular risk that comes with having type 2 diabetes.

- **Walnuts**: Walnuts are a fantastic substitute for simple carbohydrate snacks like potato chips or salted crackers since they are high in fiber, protein, and healthy fats. The fatty acids in walnuts possess the ability to not only heighten good cholesterol levels but also lower bad cholesterol. By doing this, the chance of heart disease or a heart attack may be decreased. Diabetes does heighten your risk of developing heart disease. Researchers found that those who ate nuts at least twice a week had a decreased chance of gaining weight compared to those who ate them infrequently or never at all. (Sabate, 2012) I should note that obesity and excess body fat heighten your chances of developing diabetes. For those of you who have diabetes and are still struggling with weight loss, when you start implementing certain changes and begin to lose weight, you will notice that your sugar level will improve as well. I should also note that walnuts contain fiber, and as you have been reading, you notice that fiber is great for digestion and will make you go to the bathroom healthily.

Superfoods That Are Great for Weight Loss and Management

To lose weight and maintain the weight loss you have achieved, I am in no way suggesting that you go on a starvation diet. I am in no way telling you to begin acting as if you are on a reality show and treat your kitchen as if you are in the wild with a limited source of produce. That is very extreme. What I want is for you all to eat in moderation and, more importantly, to eat smarter. I have said it before, and I will say it again: Superfoods are packed with a variety of vitamins and minerals that will not only reduce inflammation but also control your digestive tract. These two very important actions get rid of bloating, give you a lot of energy that you need to do your daily tasks, and also give you that push when working out (yes, I said working out). You also must make exercise a part of your life now.

Listed below are some (but not all) of the superfoods that are great for weight loss and management:

- **Almonds**: These nuts are great for snacking and incorporating into a fruit plate. Not only that, but studies show that people who incorporated almonds into their diet lost 62% more weight and

56% more body fat than those who decided to drop unhealthy snacks (Wein, 2003).

🌿 **Avocados**: You just cannot go wrong with avocados; they are full of potassium, which is a great way to help reduce bloating.

🌿 **Bell peppers**: Bell peppers, whether they are red, green, or yellow, are all filled with vitamins A, B2, B6, C, and E, along with potassium, dietary fiber, and folate. These are great for giving your body essential vitamins and for reducing bloating.

🌿 **Blueberries**: You know that I am a berry lover. However, the thing about blueberries that makes them stand out is that they are filled with vitamins and minerals and are a great source of fiber, which you know your body loves. The main power source of blueberries lies in their antioxidant content, which makes them one of the most powerful foods to combat pollutants and inflammation while also increasing metabolism.

🌿 **Coconut oil**: Coconut oil contains heart-healthy medium-chain triglycerides (MCT), as opposed to longer-chain triglycerides (LCT), which are the fat found in meats and dairy products. The best source of MCT is actually coconut oil. You will notice a decrease in body fat if you incorporate MCT into your lifestyle.

- **Dark chocolate**: This can help shed weight and is also very tasty. When consumed in moderation, dark chocolate contributes to weight loss and will not make you feel guilty for enjoying a healthy treat.

- **Eggs**: Eggs are a great superfood that plays an essential role in calorie cutting. Eggs contain gratifying fat and protein that control appetite. They are so versatile and can be prepared in a variety of ways! They are also excellent for muscle building (for those of you who are thinking of toning and muscle building) due to the fact that they include all nine fundamental amino acids; the more muscle you have, the more fat you burn. The yolk of an egg contains all of the fat and nearly half of the protein. It truly is nature's ideal food.

- **Grapefruit**: I made a brief mention in Chapter 4 about the grapefruit diet, and I was not encouraging you to do extreme diets. Well, what I want you to keep in mind is that a good thing to do is eat half a grapefruit before your meal, as it will assist you in not gaining any weight. This is a great aspect to keep in mind!

- **Greek yogurt**: I have mentioned that yogurt is great for your health and that you should find various ways to incorporate it into your life. It is a great source of protein, but not only that, it is great for helping to build muscle, and it keeps you full for a longer period of time, which is a good thing as it prevents overeating.

🌿 **Hazelnuts**: Those of you who buy nuts often reach for peanuts and almonds. Think about it for a second: Hazelnuts do not get as much attention as the other nuts. I am here to let you know that during my own personal experience with superfoods, eating two tablespoons of hazelnuts on a daily basis for three months, I noticed a vast improvement in my overall diet with no negative effect on my body mass index (BMI). I suggest you give it a try, make notes, and compare. If you are allergic to nuts, please do not try this.

Chapter 7

Staying Consistent and Maintaining Progress

Success is the sum of small efforts—repeated day-in and day-out.

–Robert Collier

I want you all to be healthy and improve mentally and physically. I have to draw your attention briefly to sustainability and the fact that it is an important aspect of your new superfood journey. Eating sustainably is not only beneficial to the environment but also to your overall budget and your wellness. Food must be grown in a way that preserves nature and has no negative effects on

111

biodiversity, ecosystems, or the earth's resources in order for a diet to be deemed sustainable. In addition to being safe, healthy, and socially acceptable, a diet that is environmentally friendly should be affordable. Transport-related emissions are not as harmful to the environment as emissions from food production.

I will be highlighting some ways that can help you have a more balanced and sustainable diet:

- **Consume less meat and eat more plants**: I am not in any way trying to force any of you to become vegan or vegetarian (unless that is what you wish to do). What I want to highlight is that you should aim for balance. The amount of greenhouse gas emissions associated with animal agriculture is far higher than that of vegetable protein agriculture. The manufacturing of animal feed alone results in more emissions than in the synthesis of plant-based proteins. Ultimately, the amount of food that animals need is double that of what they yield in terms of meat. Suppose you are wondering what will happen to your levels of protein if you shift how much meat you consume. Not to worry; remember that there are many products on the superfood list that are high in protein. Legumes, whole grains, nuts, and seeds are all great sources of plant-based proteins. Remember, I am not telling you to cut it out of your life; just minimize how often you consume it. Choose animal proteins such as pasteurized fish, eggs, chicken, and pork that have lower carbon emissions when making your selection. Carbon emissions from traditionally reared cattle and lamb are most prevalent, whereas the lowest emissions tend to come from beans, peas, and nuts.

- **Cut back on eating ultra-processed foods**: I am very aware that many of the changes that you wish to accomplish will not happen overnight, and it is a process. Many of you who are reading this consume processed foods in high volumes. Foods that have been highly processed usually contain a lot of fat, sugar, and additives. These are not good for any human being, and this is why it is imperative to be mindful of the levels of intake. Processed meats, chips, prepackaged desserts, and sugar-filled beverages are just a few examples of processed products. Greenhouse gas emissions become a result of the production, distribution, and consumption of these items. It is wise to reduce your intake of these processed foods, as not only your health but also the environment will benefit.

- **Be very picky when it comes to seafood**: This is one area where I will encourage being a picky eater. Current fisheries rules and regulations set forth sustainability criteria with the goals of preserving ecosystems, preventing overfishing, minimizing accidental catches, and protecting ocean habitats. One strategy used by suppliers to meet the growing demand for seafood while avoiding overfishing of the seas is aquaculture or fish breeding. This is where you may want to branch off and start eating salmon a bit more, as it will cut back on the overfishing of exotic fish and seafood. Also, those who fish for luxury, whereas you may enjoy the relaxation and joy of the catch, should also keep in mind the overall effect it has on the environment.

- **Support local businesses**: We should all make a conscious effort to choose locally grown food and produce. Selecting food that is grown nearby has the potential to lower greenhouse gas emissions, energy consumption, and resource utilization compared to when food is transported across large distances. However, if you have to travel far to acquire local goods, the advantages can be offset. My main aim is that you shop locally, wherever you can. Make an effort to look out for signs in stores that have locals in the window, and also visit local farms to get produce. Also, if you have space, consider gardening and growing your own produce. There are many self-help books that can assist you, and you will be surprised at the amazing things you accomplish.

- **Purchase your produce in season**: There are many of us who have preferences for certain produce and will not mind spending extra to purchase it out of season. Here's the thing, though: When compared to out-of-season produce, seasonal produce typically uses less fuel and produces less pollution because it travels less distance to supermarkets or stores. On the other hand, in order for produce grown outside of season to thrive, it tends to need specialized, high-energy heating and lighting. In-season produce is not only better for the environment but also frequently tastes better and costs a lot less.

🌿 **Buy in bulk**: No, I am not telling you to stock your home as if you are expecting the apocalypse. However, there are certain things that you should buy in bulk. You can cut down on unnecessary packaging waste and conserve energy and materials needed to create that packaging by buying in bulk at your local grocery store. You should invest in reusable, washable bags for your produce.

🌿 **Do your part and reduce food waste**: Food waste ends up in landfills, where it proceeds to add to air, water, and land pollution. The overall production of food also consumes a lot of energy, water, fertilizer, land, and fuel. All that for it to wind up in a landfill is a lot of resources used. So, how can you play your part in the cutback of this?

  ⯈ You can cut back on food waste by taking time to get into the habit of making meal plans. Ensure that you keep track of the food you eat.

  ⯈ Use leftovers (in the 7-day meal plan in the appendix section; this is part of it).

  ⯈ Consume all your vegetables and fruits that you purchase before they are spoiled. This is where keeping track of what you eat will be useful.

🌿 **Start practicing different recipes and make your own meals**: Preparing your own meals is another simple method to cut down on packaging waste. In addition to saving money on food manufacturing and packaging, cooking for yourself can help your overall budget as you will be cutting back on eating out or ordering food.

🌿 **Compost**: I know without a doubt that eating every last crumb of food, for instance, that peel from the apple or all your pistachio nuts, is not always a feasible task. There is not one of us who is flawless and incapable of making errors. There may be a week that you eat out or order more than you had planned. You may have forgotten your leftovers, and now they cannot be eaten as they are no longer safe to consume. You may have forgotten a particular fruit, and now it is all shriveled. Also, maybe you no longer have the desire to eat something that you set out to eat; it no longer looks appealing or attractive to you. You are a human being, and these feelings are normal. However, to prevent food from ending up in landfills, composting is a simple option. What a lovely life cycle composting creates: organic waste now becomes a nutrient-rich fertilizer that can be utilized to aid in growing more nutritious crops.

Tracking Progress and Health Benefits

I have been stressing the need to not only eat well, but you must make fitness a part of the journey. Now, I am not telling you to go and run in a marathon and swim fifteen laps in a pool every day (unless that is your goal, and you are working towards it). What I do want is for you all to be active and healthy. To prevent yourself from feeling overwhelmed, I suggest that you track your progress. It keeps you on track on this new journey, and it allows you to stay focused and even check back on things you have been or have not been doing. In the beginning, you may notice how excited you are and how you cannot wait to do certain things that you listed. However, you might find that as the weeks pass, you start to lose concentration and start to stumble. At this point, adjustments are necessary to ensure program conformity and accomplish your objectives. Rather than throwing in the towel and thinking that you cannot do this, try a new tactic that will allow you to regain control and get back on track. This is where tracking your progress comes into play. Tracking your progress, despite its seeming simplicity, is an excellent tool to monitor improvements over a period of time and hold yourself responsible.

Listed below are ways to keep you on track:

- **Keep a food log**: When you are just starting, an excellent place to start would be to make notes of what, when, and how much you consume. Take a look back at your food intake after a week of tracking to determine if any adjustments can be made. It could be possible that you are overeating, undereating, consuming too little protein or carbs, or all of the above. One apparent example could be eating an excessive amount of processed or sugar-rich meals. Documenting your nutrition makes it simpler to review it later and make changes going forward. Do not look at it and begin to think that you have been failing yourself. Keep in mind that there is a way to improve. Taking a broad view may make it easier to identify some areas of weakness in your overall nutrition. In the appendix, I listed a 7-day food plan. When you are ready to try it, log how much of it you followed through with. As you continue on your superfoods journey, make it a part of your day-to-day life. You are going to need to get into the habit of prepping meals. It would be a good idea to sit down, place these meal preps in your food log, and execute.

- **Keep track of your workouts**: I am not expecting everyone to start lifting heavy weights and running 5Ks. However, you could start taking walks around your neighborhood, and you may find that you like it, so you increase your distances, etc. These should be logged. Also, for those of you who are taking the gym route and other at-home exercises with weights. Exercises that are progressive increase harder as you gain stronger. It will get harder to recall the weight you used or the number of repetitions you performed in each set as you spend more time working out at home or in the gym. So the best thing is to log your workouts and remove the element of doubt from it. When doing weight training, record the exercise done, the number of repetitions, and the total number of sets. In addition to providing, you with a solid baseline evaluation, this will allow you to reflect on your progress and set new goals for yourself in the upcoming weeks. When engaging in cardiovascular training, make an effort to record the exercise's duration, intensity, speed, and distance covered. If you begin jogging, track how long you were jogging for, and as you improve, log the number of laps you have done or the distance.

- **Start taking progress pictures**: We see ourselves all the time. We are so used to ourselves that we will not notice certain changes. Sometimes, it is someone else who tells us we look different. As you begin this journey with the superfood way of eating. There are going to be physical changes in your body. To keep track of the great improvement, you should take photos; this will enable you to monitor your physical development.

- **Keep a weight log**: If you intend to get to a healthy weight, this is a great way to do so. You can simply record weekly weight fluctuations or select a target weight. To mark your progress, you can use a piece of paper, create a note on your phone, or go really high-tech and use an app that lets you add text to your photos. Your progress photos will show you improvements over time as well as how your body composition varies at different body weights if you include the date and your weight. When you weigh yourself, keep in mind that the number on the scale may not necessarily represent your overall health. If you are being consistent and eating right, do not freak out if the scale says you gained a pound. Also, remember that gaining muscle will reflect on the scale, but that does not mean you are gaining weight. There are many people who have unhealthy associations with a scale, and they let it control how they feel about themselves. Please, I beseech you all to keep in mind that a number on the scale does not represent your value as a person; you are more valuable than that. You can measure changes that might not be apparent to the unaided eye by using the scale as a tool. Additionally, you may notice changes in your body based on how your clothes now fit.

Superfoods to Help Your Skin Glow

Who does not want their skin to glow? There are many factors that can affect how our skin feels and looks. The truth is that the foods you eat on a regular basis have a direct impact on your skin. In fact, the foods you eat can make the difference between having tired, dull skin, which nobody wants and having a youthful, radiant complexion, which is the ultimate goal for most people. What foods, then, should you be eating to get the healthiest skin possible? Studies indicate that specific foods—specifically superfoods—will support good skin. These superfoods are powerful sources of nutrients that will nourish your skin and body from the inside out.

So let us have a look at the superfoods that will give your skin the ultimate glow-up:

- **Chia seeds**: Chia seeds will make your skin pop! A small pinch of these microseeds will give you an extra dose of omega-3 fatty acids. Here is a fun fact for you: The foundation of normal skin cell function is omega-3 fatty acids. Another key thing to note is that omega-3s aid in the synthesis of collagen. Skin strength and the battle against aging symptoms are both dependent on collagen. Chia seeds have been shown in studies to improve circulation and lessen dryness and irritation. A serving of chia seeds can work wonders for your skin. Chia seeds can be added to porridge, smoothies, or even a salad. Whichever way you choose to make them a part of your meals, just know that, along with the other amazing things it can do, it will make your skin radiate!

- **Avocados**: Avocados are just filled with so many benefits. Add benefits for your skin to the list. They are rich in mono- and polyunsaturated fatty acids. The amazing benefits of avocados are that they soothe redness and irritation and keep your skin moisturized and firm. Avocado has also been demonstrated to help shield the skin from UV rays, and if you were not aware, UV rays are a major contributor to the aging process of the skin. It also helps to maintain the suppleness and moisture retention of your skin while combating free radicals. This superfood is particularly good for those of you who have dry skin.

🌿 **Sweet potatoes**: Sweet potatoes are a wonderful source of vitamins, minerals, and fiber. They also contain beta-carotene, and this is important as the body uses it to produce vitamin A. Baked sweet potatoes have enough beta-carotene in just one half-cup serving to supply more than six times the daily recommended amount of vitamin A! How amazing is that? When ingested, beta-carotene functions as a natural sunscreen by shielding your skin cells from UV radiation. This may lessen the chance of sunburn and dry, wrinkled skin. Furthermore, studies have indicated that a rich beta-carotene diet contributes to the warm, orange tone of the skin, giving it the appearance of healthy, glowing skin. You will be glowing naturally!

🌿 **Salmon**: Omega-3s are abundant in oily fish, especially salmon. And like avocado and chia seeds, salmon helps moisturize the skin, repair damage, and keep pollutants away. Astaxanthin, which is another antioxidant found in salmon, has been demonstrated to shield skin from aging and promote younger-looking skin. This made me excited when I learned this. Having your skin look younger is always a great thing. I believe it is safe to say that most people want to age gracefully and have healthy-looking skin.

🌿 **Paprika**: The next time you are strolling in the spice aisle of the supermarket, pick up some paprika. This very bright red spice is well-known for its flavor and is used all over the world. But it is also packed with minerals, iron, fiber, and vitamins A, E, and B6, and these are all great for your skin. Sprinkle a bit over your sweet potatoes, chicken breast, eggs, rice, and a host of other foods, and you will see how the taste dances in your mouth. Papaya tastes fantastic. If you are looking for spice to give your food an extra kick while also making your skin look great, then paprika is for you.

🌿 **Spinach**: I know you are not trying to be Popeye the Sailor Man, but spinach does your body and skin good. Vitamins A, C, and K, which strengthen the skin's natural barrier and aid in the healing process after UV damage and even scarring, are quite abundant in spinach and other leafy greens like kale and collard greens. Let me break down what each of these vitamins does for your skin.

> 🌿 **Vitamin A**: This vitamin encourages moisturized, youthful, and healthy skin.

> 🌿 **Vitamin C**: This vitamin brightens your skin and evens out your skin tone.

> 🌿 **Vitamin K**: This vitamin heals scars and discolored areas and even treats under-eye circles.

Making spinach a part of your diet will lower inflammation and even prevent breakouts. Strong antioxidants found in it can also shield the skin from outside elements. It turns out that Popeye and your parents were right when they told you to eat your greens!

- ☘ **Blueberries**: They are little, but they are full of power. Blueberries pack a powerful punch in terms of skincare advantages. These very delicious berries contain a lot of antioxidants. These chemicals aid in the battle against free radicals that cause accelerated aging and damage to cells. Additionally, this fruit has been connected to enhanced circulation and heart health, both of which are critical for good skin. Consuming a cup of blueberries daily can enhance your body's capacity to deliver oxygen and nutrients to your skin and cells. This ultimately results in giving you healthier skin by enabling a faster and more effective cell turnover rate. But blueberries' health advantages don't end there. According to studies, they naturally increase collagen and may help reduce the inflammation that eczema, psoriasis, and acne cause. And you wonder why I am such a blueberry fan!

- ☘ **Lemons**: You should start incorporating lemon slices into a glass of water from now on, as it offers many skin advantages in addition to a refreshing flavor. Lemons are well-known for their purifying properties and are an excellent source of vitamin C, which is an essential vitamin for healthy skin. In addition to its role in collagen formation, vitamin C has antioxidant qualities. You can prevent and repair UV damage by including it in your diet and applying it topically (for example, by using a vitamin C serum). It has also been linked to a decreased chance of skin dryness and wrinkles. Therefore, it is a vital component in the anti-aging game.

- **Almonds**: Almonds are not only healthy snacks for your body, but they are great for your skin as well. Fiber, protein, good fats, and vitamin E are just a few of the nutrients that are abundant in these scrumptious nuts. As beneficial as almonds are for your general health, vitamin E is the star element here as it pertains to your skin. In addition to having anti-inflammatory qualities, this potent antioxidant fights the damaging effects of free radicals. It even has the ability to lessen dermatitis symptoms and sun damage to your skin. You can add some walnuts to the mixture if you want a little bit of variation. Omega-3 and omega-6 fatty acids, as well as zinc—which your skin needs to act as a barrier—are abundant in walnuts. Zinc can also aid in the fight against inflammation and germs.

- **Turmeric**: The body's inflammatory response can have a negative effect on your skin by making it appear swollen and fatigued. This can contribute to your skin aging earlier than you want, and we are not about that. But all hope is not lost because there are nutrients that can help fight this inflammation, like turmeric. This vibrant yellow-orange spice, known as turmeric, is used in many households and is packed with many benefits. Let's not forget that it is related to ginger owing to its anti-inflammatory and antioxidant qualities; it's renowned for enhancing your skin's natural radiance. In addition to supporting collagen and skin tissue, turmeric may even aid with acne scarring. Turmeric can be consumed in a variety of ways besides supplements. Try it in a tasty turmeric latte, on rice, or combined into a smoothie. Your skin will appreciate you trying out some new recipes. I have been making it a point to let you all know that it is best to explore different recipes with these ingredients. You can even mix your own turmeric face mask; there are many tutorials online that you can follow if you are interested in going that route.

- **Dark chocolate**: Yes, dark chocolate made it on the good-for-your-skin list! I can almost bet that you did not expect to see it here. Everybody occasionally needs a little dessert, and dark chocolate is a fantastic way to indulge your sweet appetite and take care of your skin at the same time. It lessens the roughness, scaling, and sunburn sensitivity of your skin.

I will leave you with this: For years, you may have been told that beauty comes from within. After reading this, you can say that it really does originate from within. Eating these superfoods will not only transform you inside but they will do wonders for your outward appearance as well. Nothing is wrong with taking care of your skin and getting that glow! Have fun experimenting with these superfoods and coming up with inventive methods to include them in your diet.

Eat These Superfoods and Watch Them Make Your Hair Healthy

Just like eating certain foods can do wonders for your skin, eating a well-balanced diet full of fish, different proteins, cereals, and other foods has a great impact on your hair, however, even though you may be aware of this information. You may not be aware of which ones to eat. If you want to learn more and discover what to eat and how it can help your hair become healthier, continue reading to learn about the superfoods you should include in your diet that will do wonders for your hair!

- **Salmon**: Omega-3 fatty acids are abundant in salmon, and they are essential for maintaining healthy scalp tissue. When these vital fatty acids are lacking, they may cause your scalp to become dry, and what this does is make the hair appear lifeless, and no one wants lifeless hair. It is crucial to pay extra attention to maintaining the health of your scalp, especially during the winter, as this is the time when your skin and hair are more susceptible to dryness.

- **Oysters**: Oysters are more known for being aphrodisiacs, so they are more than likely the last thing that comes to mind when you are thinking about hair improvement. However, they also contain zinc, which is a potent antioxidant that is necessary for strong, healthy hair and scalps. There are people who are allergic to shell food, so oysters are not for them, and there are also some people who do not fancy the taste of it. Not to worry, though; you can still give your hair the zinc it needs from beef, lamb, pumpkin seeds, and chickpeas.

- **Dark green vegetables**: Dark greens are always going to make the list! Spinach, broccoli, and Swiss chard, a leafy green vegetable commonly used in Mediterranean food preparation, are excellent providers of vitamins A and C. Your body, which depends on these vitamins, produces sebum, a greasy substance that your hair follicles naturally use to condition it. So it is great to eat up your dark green vegetables.

- **Beans**: Beans provide a great benefit for your hair that many of you may not know. You might be surprised to learn that beans, such as kidney beans, lentils, and legumes, contain protein that stimulates the growth of hair. I do not know about you, but that is great news! Some of you may be looking at different ways to gain some hair length; maybe you should give beans a try. Additionally, they are rich providers of biotin, zinc, and iron.

- **Poultry**: Turkey and chicken are excellent sources of high-quality protein. Protein does more than prevent muscle loss and maintain a healthy weight. Protein will also help to nourish and strengthen your hair. If you are not mindful, your hair may become fragile or brittle if your diet is lacking in protein, and a severe shortage of protein may cause color loss from your hair, which in turn will make it look dry and dull.

- **Nuts**: Nuts are great snacks, and they are good for your skin and your hair. Almonds, walnuts, and cashews are great sources of zinc. Zinc, as I have highlighted, is in beans and promotes hair growth. It is also found in nuts, which is good news for you. Also, if you do not get enough zinc, you might notice that you shed your hair excessively.

- **Low-fat dairy**: Low-fat dairy products with minimal fat content, which include yogurt and skim milk, are rich in protein and can help you grow healthy hair. And this is the direction that most of you want, I am sure. You cannot go wrong with healthy hair. Additionally, they contain a lot of calcium, which is a mineral that is crucial for hair development. Take some time and make Greek yogurt a part of your diet. There are many ways you can have it, and not only will it boost your health, but it will also boost your hair growth.

- **Whole grains**: Most people enjoy or rather prefer, making sandwiches with white bread because they love how it tastes. Health-wise, though, the best route is whole-grain bread. Taking the time and making this change to your eating patterns will boost your health and the overall look of your hair. Whole-grain bread, for example, is filled with zinc, iron, and vitamin B. Your hair will appreciate the added boost, and you will appreciate how your hair looks! Also, whole-grain snacks also give you a kick of energy, and who does not love added energy to make it through a long and rough day?

- **Eggs**: You just cannot go wrong with eggs, as they are a great source of protein. The aspect of eggs that I adore the most is how versatile they are in preparation; therefore, it is virtually impossible to become bored with them. Aside from that, making them a part of your diet will do great things for your hair health! This is because eggs contain biotin and vitamin B12.

- **Carrots**: Carrots are packed with benefits that are not only beneficial to your scalp but also promote good vision. This is due to the fact that carrots have an abundance of vitamin A. Take a minute and just think about it. I bet your eyes are fluttering because they are excited about these improvements, but your hair is even more exciting as it is about to become more vibrant! Take some time, add them to your salads, and make them your new snacks. Yes, I said snacks.

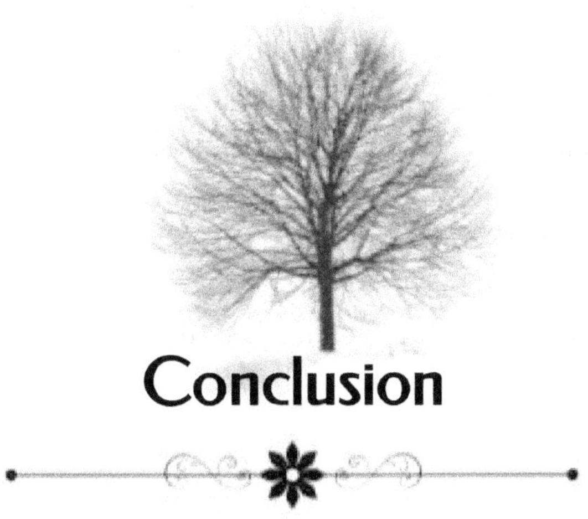

Conclusion

Wellness is the complete integration of body, mind, and spirit – the realization that everything we do, think, feel, and believe has an effect on our state of well-being.

–Greg Anderson

Superfoods Benefits Recap

I want to spend this time in this final chapter doing a recap. Leaving these reminders will reinforce the knowledge you gained from reading my book.

- **Superfoods boost your immune system**: I am not a fan of getting the cold or the flu, and I am sure none of you are. Unfortunately, it is almost impossible not to get sick at some point. We are constantly exposed to bacteria, various germs, and viruses. Our bodies are quite resilient, though, and oftentimes, they protect us from various things. However, one way to keep our immune system protected and potent is by making it our duty to consume superfoods that contain various vitamins that boost our immune system. For example, foods high in vitamins A, C, and E include citrus fruits, broccoli, almonds, and sunflower seeds. These nutrients are vital for both sustaining and bolstering our immune systems. Don't forget these superfoods, as they will make your immune system leap with joy:

- Citrus fruits (lemons, oranges)
- Ginger
- Tea (green and black)
- Nuts (almonds, cashews, walnuts)
- Sweet Potatoes
- Fatty Fish (salmon, herring, and tuna)
- Yogurt
- Poultry (chicken, turkey)
- Seeds (sunflower, chia, pumpkin)
- Beans (red, black pinto)

Superfoods help maintain your blood sugar levels: Remember when I discussed the benefits that superfoods can have for people with diabetes? Let me recap: Aside from medications that you have been prescribed by your doctor to help with your diabetes. Anyone with diabetes has to follow a specific meal plan to maintain healthy blood sugar levels. In fact, not just people with diabetes but all of us must ensure that we maintain a healthy blood sugar level. Foods that are great for keeping your blood sugar level in check:

- Tomatoes
- Seeds (pumpkin and flax)
- Turmeric
- Whole grains (oats and barley)
- Mixed nuts
- Beans (Lima, kidney and black)
- Fish (tuna, salmon, mackerel)
- Lentils
- Greek yogurt

- **Superfoods can help you on your weight management and loss journey**: Remember that the real key to losing weight in a healthy manner and maintaining it is not by eating little to nothing and living in constant hunger. Let's be honest, you will be very miserable and annoyed. The best approach is to eat in moderation and fill your plate with healthy food that will leave you energized and full. This is where superfoods come in to save the day. Superfoods such as spinach, watermelon, tomatoes, bell peppers, sweet potatoes, and salmon are rich in nutrients including, protein, potassium, vitamin C, and omega-3s, which can play a huge role in reducing your appetite, diminishing hunger levels, and helping with building muscle mass. Here are some reminders of some superfoods that can help with weight loss:

- Tomatoes
- Spinach
- Watermelon
- Seeds (chia, flax)
- Apples
- Sweet potatoes
- Chickpeas
- Dark chocolate
- Oats
- Eggs

Superfoods can help with lowering bad cholesterol levels: Not eating well and using certain oils to cook meals can increase your cholesterol levels. Having high cholesterol levels makes you more vulnerable to heart issues. When you make superfoods a part of your life, they will lower bad cholesterol levels. Superfoods are packed with monounsaturated fats and fiber, two amazing nutrients that are great for lowering bad cholesterol. Here are some superfoods that are great for lowering bad cholesterol levels:

- Apples

- Spinach

- Avocados

- Beans

- Cashews

- Goji berries

- Celery

- Fish

- **Superfoods can lower your blood pressure**: There are 1.13 billion people worldwide who suffer from hypertension, according to the World Health Organization (WHO). This is, without a doubt, a serious medical condition. However, if you are someone who is concerned about getting hypertension, by embracing superfoods and consuming foods that are packed with potassium, magnesium, and fiber, you can help reduce and prevent the risk of developing high blood pressure. Here are some superfoods that can help with the lowering of your blood pressure:

  - Berries

  - Bananas

- Beets

- Dark chocolate

- Kiwis

- Oats

- Watermelon

- Garlic

- Greek yogurt

- Cinnamon

- Pistachios

- Pomegranate

Top Five Things to Keep in Mind When Embarking on Your New Superfood Lifestyle

- **Colors are your new best friend**: Fruits and vegetables have so many different ranges of colors. They are so vibrant and filled with many lovely smells and flavors. To enhance the variety of micronutrients in your diet, try to eat as many different-colored fruits and vegetables as you can. It will keep you interested and excited.

- **You cannot get enough fiber**: Fiber is a great asset to our bodies and serves many purposes. Not only does it keep us full, but fiber promotes digestive health and may aid in weight loss. Replacing white bread and spaghetti with whole-grain equivalents is a simple method to increase your intake of fiber. You can enhance your intake of fiber by consuming whole grains and nuts.

🌿 **Watch your cholesterol intake**: There are many times you may consume high levels of cholesterol. Remember that there are superfoods that will bring your cholesterol levels down. Also, switch out the kinds of oils you cook with and invest in olive oil and coconut oil.

🌿 **Minimize your salt intake**: I am going to make this short and sweet. High levels of salt are linked to an increase in high blood pressure.

🌿 **Monitor how much sugar you consume**: There are many fruits that have natural sugar that you can get from them by consuming superfoods. Remember to avoid those ultra-processed foods, as they are loaded with sugar. High levels of sugar intake can lead to health complications like diabetes.

Superfoods to Boost Your Brain Power

Remember these superfoods while you're considering methods to sharpen and develop your cognitive abilities. You only have one brain, so be sure you're giving it the care it needs:

- **Avocados**: They are so versatile and delicious, and they are good for you. Along with all their other benefits, they are good for promoting blood flow to your brain and keeping your brain healthy.

- **Blueberries**: I promise I am not just adding this on here because I have a berry bias. They do possess antioxidants that fight off cognitive deterioration.

- **Coffee**: Coffee is a true drink of champions. The healthiest way to consume coffee is black. However, if that is too hardcore for you, instead of using sugar, use honey. Coffee can affect the processing, memory, and focus levels of your brain.

- **Dark chocolate**: This delicious treat not only aids with weight loss but is great for your brain! It possesses antioxidants that boost your brain power. Please do not binge-eat dark chocolate now; remember, everything must be done in moderation.

- **Nuts and seeds**: From almonds to walnuts, flax to chia seeds. These superfoods are great for boosting your brain's function. These are the snacks that you should have in your pantry from now on.

- **Sage**: No, I am not telling you to clear out spirits from your home. However, this herb is great for boosting your memory.

- **Turmeric**: This colorful spice can not only boost your mood but your memory as well.

- **Wild salmon**: Fish are great brain food. Wild salmon promotes healthy brain function.

I enjoyed sharing my deep passion and enthusiasm with you about superfoods. I hope that there is something that connects with you and that you find that you are ready to take that step into nurturing your body the way that it deserves. What I want you to keep in mind is that you should always ensure that you are patient with yourself, and that no aspect of this change will occur overnight. So do not be frustrated if you slip up. As you embark on this new healthy lifestyle, the most important thing is that you dust yourself off and try again. This is a lifelong journey, not a quick fix. This is officially your new path.

The important thing is that you take the time to find the superfoods that work for you and try out new recipes. There are so many options and a barrage of recipes that you will not get bored. I also do not want you to go out and try five million different things at once and then start feeling overwhelmed and no longer want to keep at this.

Take your time, start small, and work your way up. You can create your own level, and at each level, you set a particular goal, and then you move on to the next level. What I want you all to keep in mind is that you are in control. Do not compare yourself to anyone other than yourself. We are all not structured the same; we all have our own personal hurdles to overcome. So, do not ever feel that you are not getting something right based on someone else's journey. Do not ever feel as if you cannot do this. Because you can, your body will appreciate it, and you will be thankful that you did this for yourself and your body. One day, you will look back and realize how far you came and how many benefits came along with it. I believe in all of you.

Chapter "Good Will"

You have the power to make a huge impact on someone else's life and help them step towards a future of true fulfillment. All it takes is a few words.

Simply by sharing your honest opinion of this book and a little about your own story, you'll show new readers where they can find all the guidance they need to set forth on the path toward their best life.

Helping others without expectation of anything in return has been proven to lead to increased happiness and satisfaction in life.

I would love to give you the chance to experience that same feeling during your reading or listening experience today...

All it takes is a few moments of your time to answer one simple question:

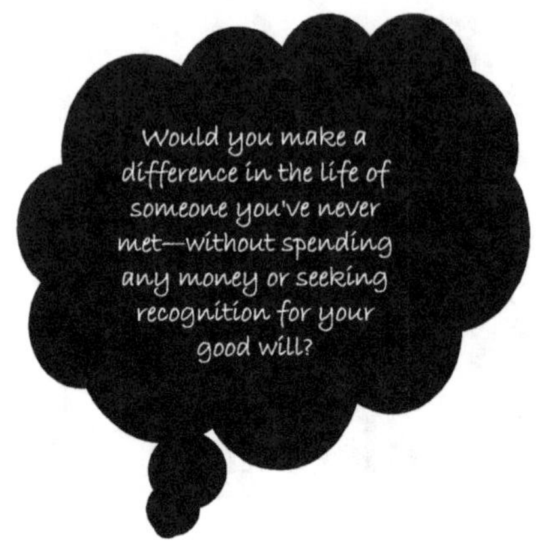

If so, then here is my small request from you again.

If you've found value in your reading or listening experience today, I humbly ask that you take a brief moment right now to leave an honest review of this book. It won't cost you anything but 30 seconds of your time—just a few seconds to share your thoughts with others.

Your voice can go a long way in helping someone else find the same inspiration and knowledge that you have.

Are you familiar with leaving a review for an Audible, Kindle, or e-reader book? If so, it's simple:

If you're on **Audible**: just hit the three dots in the top right of your device, click rate & review, then leave a few sentences about the book along with your star rating.

If you're reading on **Kindle** or an e-reader, simply scroll to the last page of the book and swipe up—the review should prompt from there.

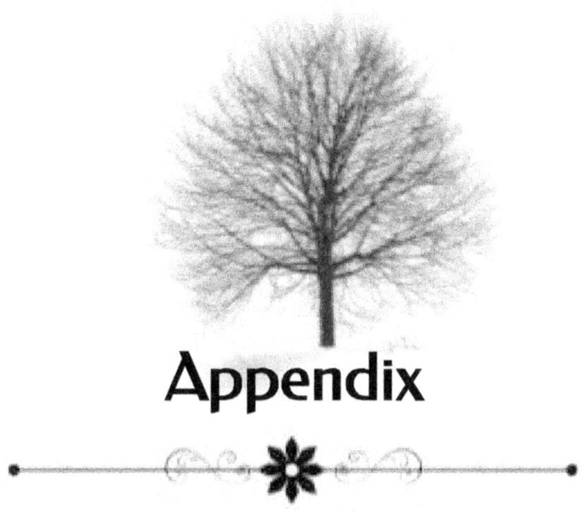

Appendix

Day 1

Breakfast

Try out a nice avocado egg sandwich. Between 2 slices of whole wheat bread (up to you if you want to toast it or not), place 1 egg and 1/4 slice of avocado. Add more color to your sandwich and place 1 slice of tomato. Enjoy that nutritious packed breakfast, and do not forget to add fruit (1 orange).

Snack

1 ounce of walnuts

Lunch

Go for a salmon salad sandwich. Trust me, this is delicious!

What you will need to do is mix fresh salmon that has been cooked. Or if you do not have that, you can mix 6 ounces of canned salmon with mashed avocado. You will need 1 tablespoon of diced red onions and 1/4 teaspoon of dill. Spread some of the mix between two slices of whole wheat bread, top it off with 1/4 cup of spinach, and enjoy! You can save the remaining salad mix for leftovers.

Snack

1 cup of raspberries, or you can opt for 1 cup of sliced cucumbers with 1 ounce of goat cheese.

Dinner

- Chicken paillard (pan-fried and easy to serve)
- You are going to need olive oil
- 2 red peppers; they should be sliced and seeded
- 1 clove of garlic should be peeled and thinly sliced
- 2 anchovies that are roughly chopped
- A small bunch of flat-leaf parsley that is roughly chopped
- 1/2 lemon
- 2 skinless chicken breast fillets

Heat your pan, place the garlic, peppers, onion, and anchovies, and let them fry for 5 minutes. Then place the chicken in it, squeeze the lemon over it, add extra peppers and parsley, and enjoy.

Day 2

Breakfast

Salmon toast. Remember the salmon mix left over from yesterday? Today will be your breakfast meal. This cuts back on prep time for you. You can have a cup of blueberries with your breakfast.

Lunch

Your leftover chicken paillard and you can have this with 1/2 can of chickpeas

Snack

Mediterranean power snack: 1 cup of grape tomatoes, 5 olives, and 1 ounce of goat cheese. Enjoy this filling snack as you continue through your day, and do not forget to stay hydrated and drink water.

Dinner

- Yacon, spinach, and watercress salad

- Chop each of the ingredients listed in a bowl and place them in a bowl.

- Your leftover chickpeas should be added to this mix along with 1 hard-boiled egg

- 1/2 ounce goat cheese

- 1/3 ounce of walnuts

- 1 1/2 tablespoons of lemon juice (optional)

🌿 Mixed with 2 teaspoons of olive oil

Day 3

Breakfast

Smoothie! You can try this blended oat smoothie. You can pick your berry of choice. In a blender, combine 1/4 cup of oats, 1/2 teaspoon of maqui powder (optional), and 1 cup of berries. Add ice and blend! Have an apple with your smoothie.

Lunch

Wild sardine toasts. On two slices of whole wheat toast, place sardines, 1/2 ounce of goat cheese, along with 1/4 teaspoon of lemon zest, and enjoy!

Snack

1 cup of berries and a handful of almonds

Dinner

Lazy day beef and vegetable soup: This is good if you are not in the mood to stand and cook. If this process is too long, you can draw from a previous recipe.

🌿 2 1/2 pounds of beef stew meat, cut into chunks

🌿 2 cans of reduced-sodium beef broth

🌿 1 can chickpeas, rinsed and drained

🌿 Estimate diced tomatoes

- 1 cup of water

- 1/2 teaspoon salt

- 1/2 teaspoon pepper

- 2 cups mixed vegetables (peas, carrots, corn, and green beans)

- 1 cup of uncooked small pasta

Combine beef, broth, chickpeas, tomatoes, water, salt, and pepper in a quart slow cooker; toss to coat well. Cover and cook on high for five hours. (No repeated stirring is necessary during this process). Proceed to add your mixed vegetables and pasta. Continue cooking, covered, for about an hour or until your beef and pasta are tender. Season with salt and pepper, as desired. Stir well before serving.

Day 4

Breakfast

Make some nice apple-cinnamon oatmeal.

Cook 1/2 cup oats in 1 cup water with 1 chopped apple; stir in 1 tablespoon of chia seeds, chopped walnuts, and 1/8 teaspoon of cinnamon. Enjoy with a slice of grapefruit.

Lunch

Enjoy your lazy beef stew from yesterday. You can even have it with a slice of whole-wheat bread.

Snack

Berries and Greek yogurt mix

- 1 cup raspberries with 1/2 cup of yogurt and 1 tablespoon of ground flaxseeds

Dinner

Pan-fry 4-ounce pork in 1/2 teaspoon of olive oil with 1 clove of garlic and 1/2 teaspoon rosemary.

- Also, add 2 cups broccoli, sautéed in 1 tsp

- Olive oil with 1 clove of garlic

- And add 1 sweet potato, baked

Pan-fry all the ingredients listed according to your taste preference. Enjoy with your baked sweet potato and broccoli.

Day 5

Breakfast

Another smoothie morning! Almond Pear Smoothie

In your blender, proceed to combine 1 cup kefir, 1 pear, chopped, 1 tablespoon almond butter, and ice, and then blend. Enjoy with mango slices!

Snack

Fruit mix! Combine your favorite fruits from the superfoods list and make a nice fruit bowl with water.

Lunch

Salad wrap. Get spinach or whole wheat wrap. Place lettuce, carrots, tomatoes, and cucumbers in the wrap. Locate a low-calorie salad dressing or top it with 1 ounce of goat cheese and enjoy.

Snack

Fruit mix! Combine your favorite fruits from the superfoods list and make a nice fruit bowl with water.

Dinner

Pan-fried Pork Leftovers

Snack

3/4 cup of fruit mixed yogurt

Day 6

Breakfast

I did not forget the eggs! Mushroom and spinach omelet

What you will need to do is sauté 3 tablespoons of chopped mushrooms and 1/2 cup baby spinach with garlic powder. Add 2 eggs, whisked. When you notice your eggs begin to set, add 1/2 ounce of goat cheese. Cook until set. Enjoy with 1 cup of raspberries.

Lunch

Red and green smoothie. Yes, sometimes it is nice to mix things up!

Proceed to blend. 1 cup kefir, 1/2 cup yogurt, 2 cups spinach, 1 cup of berries (your choice), 1/2 cup seeded and chopped cucumber, and 1/4 cup oats. Add ice, blend, and enjoy.

Snack

1/2 cup of grape tomatoes

Dinner

- Tuna power salad
- 1 cup cooked Farro (optional)
- 1 can tuna packed in water (prefer if you get tuna fresh and cook it)
- 3/4 cup grape tomatoes, sliced in half
- 1/4 cup green olives, sliced in half
- 1/4 cup walnuts, toasted and coarsely chopped
- 1/4 cup shaved Parmesan cheese
- 1/4 cup fresh basil, sliced into thin strips
- 2 tablespoons of olive oil

Salt and pepper to taste for added flavor.

Place all the ingredients on a platter above. Finish with droplets of olive oil and a sprinkling of salt and pepper to taste. This meal is best served at room temperature. You can keep leftovers in your refrigerator for up to 3 days and they are best served at room temperature.

Day 7

Breakfast

Monkey Toast. Place two slices of toasted whole wheat bread with 2 tablespoons of almond butter and 1/2 banana, sliced. Enjoy this breakfast meal with 3/4 cup of yogurt and an orange.

Lunch

- Spicy black bean tacos
- 1 tablespoon of olive oil
- 3 garlic cloves, sliced thinly
- 2 cans of black beans, drained and rinsed
- 3 tablespoons of cider vinegar
- 1 1/2 tablespoons honey
- 1 1/2 tablespoons ground cumin
- For the guacamole
- 1 small garlic clove
- 2 tablespoons roughly chopped coriander
- 1 green chili, sliced
- 2 avocados (mashed)
- Lime juice

- For the salsa

- 110-gram pack of pomegranate seeds

- 1 green chili, finely diced

- 1 finely diced white onion

Place all the ingredients together and cook and place honey and other spices in to add flavor.the

When ready to eat. Place the mix in vegetable tortillas with hot sauce (optional) and coconut yogurt.

Dinner

Leftover tuna power salad!

Snack

Air-popped popcorn

Superfood Recipes You Can Try

The variety makes this journey exciting! Add your own twist to the recipes if you like, try them, and see what works for your taste buds!

Raspberry Chicken Lettuce Wraps

These wraps are creative and packed with a nice flavor! They are also easy to put together.

- 1/4 cup of raspberry preserve

- 2 tablespoons of olive oil

- 1 tablespoon of white wine vinegar

- 1 teaspoon of mustard

- Salt and fresh ground pepper

- 2 tablespoons minced scallions

- 1 cup of fresh raspberries

- 4 cooked chicken breast halves, cut into 1-inch pieces

- 4 cups of chopped lettuce

Directions

Get yourself a nice-sized bowl and whip together the raspberry preserves, oil, vinegar, mustard, and salt and pepper. You should then proceed to add scallions and raspberries to the vinaigrette. Add diced chicken and toss to combine with the vinaigrette. Arrange the lettuce on plates however you want them arranged. Then proceed to add the chicken mixture over the lettuce and chow down!

Tomato and Barley Soup

This recipe is perfect for days when you want to make a quick, easy, and tasty soup. The great thing about this menu is that you will have leftovers.

- 1 cup of diced onions

- 1 cup of diced carrots

- 1 cup of diced celery

- 2 teaspoons of minced garlic

- 2 tablespoons of olive oil

- 1/3 cup barley

- 1 (14-ounce) can stewed tomatoes

- 2 cups chicken broth

- 2 cups of water

- 1 bay leaf

- 1/8 teaspoon of black pepper

Directions

You are going to need a medium to large-sized pot to make this tasty soup. In your pot, heat the olive oil and proceed to add the onions, carrots, celery, and garlic. Let it sauté for about 10 minutes or until the vegetables start to soften. While this is happening pour the barley into a dish with water to cover. Proceed to add the tomatoes, broth, water, bay leaf, and pepper and bring to a boil, you should stir this occasionally. Drain the barley and add to the pot. Reduce heat and cook at a low boil for about 45 minutes, or until barley is tender. If you notice that it is thickening too much, proceed to add water.

Healthy Oatmeal and Apple Muffins

Of course, I had to dig up a muffin recipe for you! You can have a tasty snack, and it will be healthy!

- 1 1/2 cup quick oats

- 1 1/2 cup apple juice

- 2 teaspoons of vanilla extract

- 1 1/2 cup whole wheat flour

- 1/2 cup of honey

- 2 teaspoons baking powder

- 2 medium apples (they are going to need to be grated)

- 1 teaspoon cinnamon

- 4 egg whites, beaten

- Apple wedges for garnish (it is fine, with or without the peel)

Directions

You are going to need to soak the oats, apple juice, honey, and vanilla together for 30 minutes. Then, mix in the flour, baking powder, grated apple, and cinnamon. After mixing all those ingredients, add the egg whites. Get out your muffin tins and start placing the mix in the tins. Proceed to top the muffins with the apple wedges. You should bake your muffins at 170 °C (338 °F) for 25–30 minutes until the muffins are done and have a nice golden color. Allow them to cool for a few minutes, and then remove your lovely fluffy muffin from the rack and enjoy. I don't know about you, but my mouth is watering!

Blueberry Banana Pancakes

I had to add a breakfast recipe to the list. It is always great to make a nice, healthy breakfast that everyone will enjoy!

- 1 cup skim milk (or you could use almond milk or the milk that you normally use)

- 1 tablespoon vinegar or 1 tablespoon lemon juice

- 1/2 cup whole wheat flour

- 1 tablespoon Splenda sugar substitute

- 1 1/2 teaspoon baking powder

- 1/2 teaspoon salt

- 1/4 teaspoon nutmeg

- 2 egg whites

- 2 tablespoons oil

- 1 banana, mashed

- 3/4 cup of blueberries, preferably fresh. However, if you only have frozen food, that's fine.

Directions

Once you have gathered all your ingredients, proceed to pour the vinegar or lime juice into the milk and let it sit for five minutes. After doing that, mix all the dry ingredients together in a bowl: whole wheat flour, baking powder, etc.

After doing that, proceed to stir the milk/vinegar mixture, then mix the egg whites, oil, and banana together.

After doing that, it is time for you to pour the liquid mix into the dry mix and stir until it is well blended. You should not try to overmix it. If you notice that your batter is a bit too thick, get some more milk and add it; this will help to thin it out a bit.

Heat your griddle or frying pan to medium heat. Proceed to grease the griddle or pan and then add 1/4 cup of batter to it. Take this time to place the blueberries on the pancake. Cook until golden to medium brown. Serve with sliced bananas or syrup and enjoy.

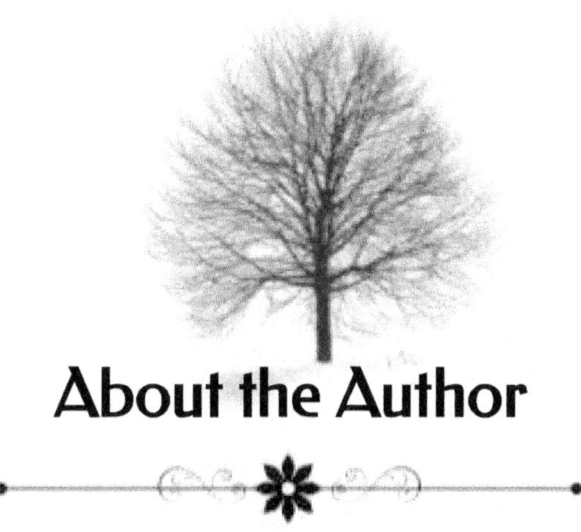

About the Author

This author has a knack for capturing the essence of life's complexities, intricacies, and universal truths through her writing, often presenting thought-provoking perspectives on various aspects of existence. Her life books are characterized by rich character development, as the author skillfully weaves together the stories of diverse topics, illuminating journeys, challenges, and triumphs. Through books, the author explores themes such as love, passion, victory, identity, personal growth, and the search for meaning, offering readers profound insights and moments of introspection.

Beyond Zoë's professional accomplishments, she also has a rich and multifaceted life outside of publishing. This book is a testament to her commitment to providing valuable insights and practical guidance. The author's books are often praised for their ability to evoke empathy in readers, fostering a deep connection between the readers and the valuable insights they encounter within the pages.

The author is a distinguished authority in various fields of study, bringing a wealth of knowledge and experience to her thought-provoking non-fiction works. As you delve into Zoë's manuscripts, you can expect to embark on an intellectual journey guided by Zoë's profound insights and intentional thought-provoking passion for self - development. Her non-fiction works continue to push the boundaries of knowledge, inviting readers to expand their horizons and gain a deeper understanding of life and its impact on our success.

Zoë's works have been praised for their meticulous research, insightful analysis, and the way they challenge readers to think critically about the world around them.

Any one of Zoë's latest books,....

1. Unlocking Infinity: Master the Art of Longevity

Learn How to, Boost Your Brain Health, Recharge Your Immune System and Restore Youthful Balance in 3 Easy Steps

2. Living Your Best Life: Radiate from Within

Ultimate Guide to Finding Purpose & Fulfillment in 3 Easy Steps.

3. Alone, But Not Lonely: Aging on Your Terms

A Roadmap for Aging Independently, Striking Balance & Finding Purpose

4. Redefining Aging: The Art of Living Alone

How to Find Joy in Independence, Live Fearlessly & Maintain Longevity

5. Journeying Alone, Journeying Strong: Navigating Aging Alone Without Children

Self-Help Guide to Finding Inner Strength, Peace, Joy & Fulfillment in Childless Aging

6. Mastering the Steps to Success: Achieving Success at Every Rung

Proven Strategies for Overcoming Obstacles and Reaching Greatness. Develop, Learn, Succeed

7. The Positivity Code: Supercharge Your Life with Positive Thinking

Learn The Art of Positive Thinking, Changing Your Life One Thought at a Time

8. The Growth Mindset Code: Cracking the Secrets to Success

Comprehensive Guide to Breaking Limits with A Growth Mindset, Cultivating Unlimited Possibilities

9. Longevity: The Art of Aging Backwards

Step-by-Step Guide to Renew, Restore and Reverse Aging Mentally, Physically & Spiritually

… is another testament to her dedication to delivering enlightening and captivating non-fiction literature. Whether you're a seasoned reader of non-fiction or new to the genre Zoë's work is sure to engage, inform, and inspire. To stay updated on **Zoë Publishing's** latest projects and musings, visit us on **facebook.com/zoepublishing** and follow us on ….

Instagram & Tik Tok **(@zoepublishing)**

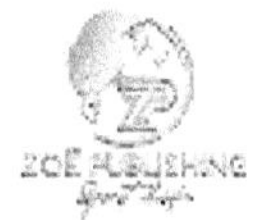

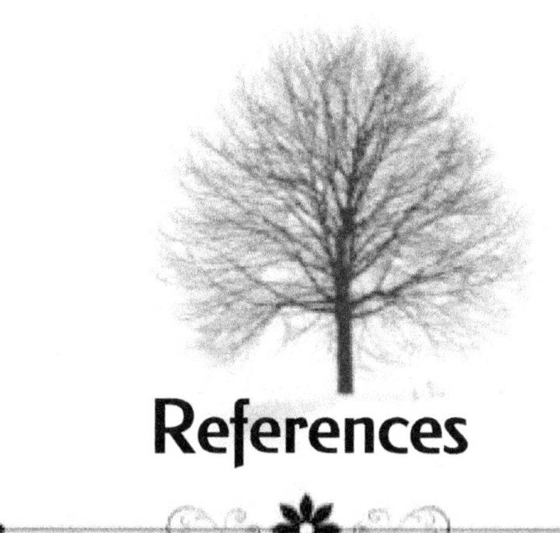

References

Bainbridge, H. (2020, November 6). *Superfoods to the rescue.* Clean Eating. https://www.cleaneatingmag.com/meal-plans/energy-boosting-meal-plans/7-day-superfoods-meal-plan/

Bainbridge H. (2016, October). *Superfood meal plan.* Clean Eating. https://cdn2.hubspot.net/hubfs/4566937/Healthy%20Living%20Group/Clean%20Eating/CE%20All-Access%20Membership/PDFs%20-%20Member%20Content%20Export/Energy-Boosting%20Meal%20Plans/Superfoods%20to%20the%20Rescue/SuperFood%20Meal%20Plan%20Copy%20.pdf

Barnes, M. (2023, September 5). *6 tips on overcoming picky eating as an adult.* The Art of Healthy Living. https://artofhealthyliving.com/6-tips-on-overcoming-picky-eating-as-an-adult/

Bastin, G. (2020, January 6). *The top 100 superfoods of 2020.* Opportuniteas. https://opportuniteas.com/blogs/news/the-top-100-superfoods

Best Superfoods to Promote Heart Health. (2022, November). Dedication Health. https://www.dedication-health.com/best-superfoods-to-promote-heart-health/

Biswas, C. (2023, July 8). *Top 24 healthy food quotes to inspire you.* Stylecraze. https://www.stylecraze.com/articles/slogans-on-healthy-food/

Burke, A. (2014, September 26). *Tracking your progress for health and fitness success.* Huffpost. https://www.huffpost.com/entry/tracking-your-progress-fo_b_5883622

Carter, N. (2023, August 3). *Teen nutrition: 5 inevitable superfoods for teenagers.* Helena Study. https://www.helenastudy.com/teen-nutrition-superfoods-for-teenagers/

Chicken paillard. (2023, May 18). Olive Magazine. https://www.olivemagazine.com/recipes/meat-and-poultry/chicken-paillard-with-red-peppers/

Finken, N. (2020, May 11). *How to eat sustainably: 10 tips for a healthy body and planet. To Taste.* https://totaste.com/eating-sustainably/

Gayla, V. (2013). *Tomato and barley soup.* Food.com. https://www.food.com/recipe/tomato-and-barley-soup-280466

George, T. (2023). *The pros and cons of adding superfood powder to your diet.* Healthy Lifestyle Blog. https://healthhub.hif.com.au/nutrition/the-pros-and-cons-of-adding-superfood-powder-to-your-diet

Gwinn, A. (2022, August 4). *8 superfoods to eat after 50.* AARP. https://www.aarp.org/health/healthy-living/info-2021/superfoods-for-adult-health.html

Herbert, J. (2020, July). *9 Superfoods for healthier digestion.* Select Health. https://selecthealth.org/blog/2020/07/9-superfoods-for-healthier-digestion

How to incorporate superfoods into everyday meals. (2023, October 8). Healthy Blog. https://foodtolive.com/healthy-blog/how-to-incorporate-superfoods-into-everyday-meals/

Improve your joint health with these 12 superfoods. (2022, June 28). Oregon Shoulder Institute. https://www.oregonshoulder.com/blog-posts/improve-your-joint-health-with-these-12-superfoods

Jokosusilo. (2023, September 30). *Eating healthy on a budget: affordable superfoods for every diet.* Medium. https://medium.com/@jokosusilo101997/eating-healthy-on-a-budget-affordable-superfoods-for-every-diet-84c48c135991

Joyce, J. (2020). *Spicy black bean tacos.* BBC Good Food. https://www.bbcgoodfood.com/recipes/spicy-black-bean-tacos

Lehmann, A. (2023, February 9). *Healthy nutrition — the science of superfood: separating fact from fiction.* Medium. https://dailyknowhow.medium.com/healthy-nutrition-the-science-of-superfood-separating-fact-from-fiction-d7a3ca44a67c

Maher, P., Dargusch, R., Ehren, J.L., Okada, K.S., Schubert, D. (2011, June 27). *Fisetin lowers methylglyoxal dependent protein glycation and limits the complications of diabetes.* PLOS One. https://journals.plos.org/plosone/article?id=10.1371/journal.pone.0021226

Majumdar, S. PhD. (2017, March 11). *7 Super foods you should definitely eat during your menstrual cycle.* Practo. https://www.practo.com/healthfeed/7-super-foods-you-should-definitely-eat-during-your-menstrual-cycle-27199/post

Manning, P.J., Sutherland, W.H., Walker, R.J., Williams, S.M., Jong, S.A., Ryalls, A.R., Berry, E.A. (2004, September 1). *Effect of high-dose vitamin e on insulin resistance and associated parameters in overweight subject.* American Diabetes Association. https://diabetesjournals.org/care/article/27/9/2166/22595/Effect-of-High-Dose-Vitamin-E-on-Insulin

McPherson, G. (2022, April 19). *How to make healthy, kid-friendly meals for picky eaters*. Healthline. https://www.healthline.com/nutrition/healthy-meals-for-picky-eaters

Melibug. (2008). *Raspberry chicken lettuce wraps*. Food. Com. https://www.food.com/recipe/raspberry-chicken-lettuce-wraps-289146#reviews

Nunez, K. (2023, February 21). *6 Exceptional superfoods to eat for a strong, healthy immune system*. Real Simple. https://www.realsimple.com/foods-for-immune-system-7093660

Phytonutrients – nature's natural defense. (2019, January 3). Unlock Food. https://www.unlockfood.ca/en/Articles/Vitamins-and-Minerals/Phytonutrients-%E2%80%93-Nature%E2%80%99s-Natural-Defense.aspx#:~:text=Many%20phytonutrients%20have%20antioxidant%20properties,stroke%2C%20Alzheimer's%20and%20Parkinson's%20disease.

Pope, J. (2022, September 15). *Evaluating dietary supplements for efficacy and safety*. Macmillan Learning. https://community.macmillanlearning.com/t5/nutrition-blog/evaluating-dietary-supplements-for-efficacy-and-safety/ba-p/17450

Reist, W. (2017, September 18). *Tuna superfood power salad*. Sweet Cayenne. https://sweetcayenne.com/tuna-superfood-power-salad/

Richmond, C. (2022, June 23). *How to overcome picky eating as an adult.* Web MD. https://www.webmd.com/food-recipes/ss/slideshow-picky-eating

Rowlings, E. (2023, July 15). *5 Amazing benefits of superfoods.* The Upside. https://www.vitacost.com/blog/benefits-of-superfoods/

Sabate, J., Rastrollo- Bes, M., Gracia- Gomez, E., Alonso, A., Gonzalez- Martinez, M.A. (2012, September 6). *Nut consumption and weight gain in a Mediterranean cohort: the SUN study.* Wiley Online Library. https://onlinelibrary.wiley.com/doi/full/10.1038/ob y.2007.507

Schultz, R. (2023). *The 15 best superfoods for weight loss.* Muscle and Fitness. https://www.muscleandfitness.com/nutrition/lose-fat/best-superfoods-weight-loss/

Shaban, D. (2023, June 26). *Health benefits of antioxidants.* Web Md. https://www.webmd.com/diet/health-benefits-antioxidants

Stanton, B. (2022). *Bioavailability and nutrient density: Optimizing your diet for more nutrition.* Carb Manager. https://www.carbmanager.com/article/y2oy0xaaa minwxtv/bioavailability-and-nutrient-density-optimizing-your

The benefits of a nutrient-dense diet. (2023, July 10). Moorings Park. https://www.mooringspark.org/news/the-benefits-of-a-nutrient-dense-diet

The truth about superfoods. (2014, August). Provitamil. https://www.provitamil.com/healthier-lifestyle/the-truth-about-superfoods.htm

Thompson, K. (2023, January 18). *15 Best superfood powders to try, according to nutrition experts.* Mind Body Green. https://www.mindbodygreen.com/articles/superfood-powders

Ware, M. (2023, August 2). *Ten diabetes superfoods.* Medical News Today. https://www.medicalnewstoday.com/articles/317112

Wein, M.A., Sabate, J.M., Ikle, N., Cole, S.R., Kandeel, F.R. (2003, November 27). *Almonds vs complex carbohydrates in a weight reduction program.* National Library of Medicine. https://pubmed.ncbi.nlm.nih.gov/14574348/

What are superfoods and are they really super? (2012, December 11). EUFIC. https://www.eufic.org/en/healthy-living/article/the-science-behind-superfoods-are-they-really-super

What is a superfood, anyway? (2021, November 10). Cleveland Clinic.

https://health.clevelandclinic.org/what-is-a-superfood/

Y. Stephanie. (2014). *Blueberry banana pancake*. Food.com. https://www.food.com/recipe/blueberry-banana-pancakes-317835#reviews

10 Super foods good for your heart. (2021). Health X Change.). https://www.healthxchange.sg/food-nutrition/food-tips/ten-superfoods-protect-heart

10 super foods for healthy hair. (2023). True Skincare Center. https://trueskincarecenter.com/blog/10-super-foods-for-healthy-hair/

10 Superfoods to boost brain power. (2019, July 9). United Brain Association. https://unitedbrainassociation.org/2019/07/09/10-superfoods-to-boost-brain-power/

11 superfoods for glowing skin. (2023, August 30). Herbal Dynamics Beauty. https://www.herbaldynamicsbeauty.com/blogs/herbal-dynamics-beauty/superfoods-for-glowing-skin

14 Balanced beef superfood recipes to try in the New Year. (2021, January 5). Beef loving Texans. https://beeflovingtexans.com/stories/14-balanced-beef-superfood-recipes-to-try-in-the-new-year/

www.ingramcontent.com/pod-product-compliance
Lightning Source LLC
Chambersburg PA
CBHW070859160726
48004CB00003B/1159